Viv Martin was just home from a family holiday in Italy when a strange tingling feeling started in the left side of her mouth. It soon spread down her left side until it reached her left hand. After visits to her GP, a referral to a neurologist, and tests in hospital, she learned she had a life-threatening neurological condition. Delicate brain surgery would ultimately be required. Completely frank and utterly moving, this is the story of how Viv Martin underwent that brain surgery – and survived.

Feeling vulnerable and powerless, she knew she had to find some means of maintaining a degree of control. For her, this meant confronting her situation as honestly as she could: by seeking a clear and complete picture of her condition, by using complementary healing, and by drawing on the support of family and friends. As she faces the possibility of dying, she reflects on the psychological and spiritual meaning of serious illness, revealing her feelings and sharing the insights she gained from her experience

Viv Martin began her career as a primary school teacher, then spent three years teaching English in a secondary school in Zambia. On returning to England she gained a B.Phil. (Ed) degree. After teaching English at secondary level for a year, she left full-time work to have her two children, and has since worked as a sessional teacher for Birmingham Tuition Service. She has also trained as a bereavement counsellor for Cruse and completed a counselling course at a local further education college, where she later worked part-time as a counsellor and teacher. As her recovery continues, she hopes to go on with work in the counselling field.

OUT OF MY HEAD

An Experience of Neurosurgery

Viv Martin

The Book Guild Ltd
Sussex, England

The Book Guild Ltd.
25 High Street
Lewes, Sussex

First published 1997
© Viv Martin, 1997
Set in Times
Typesetting by Poole Typesetting (Wessex) Ltd, Bournemouth.
Printed in Great Britain by
Athenaeum Press Ltd, Gateshead

A catalogue record for this book is
available from the British Library

ISBN 1 85776 179 0

*In memory of Margaret,
a good friend and an inspiration*

CONTENTS

ACKNOWLEDGEMENTS

I am indebted:

to my fellow patients at the Midland Centre for Neurosurgery and Neurology for all we shared.

to all the staff at MCNN, particularly the radiographers and the nurses on Ward D for their care and compassion, and to Dr Milne Anderson and Mr Carl Meyer, two very special people.

to my friends and family who gave me so much in their unique and individual ways.

to Tony for his love and support.

to Steve and Josie for being themselves.

to Val and Doris for all their help and support.

to the healers, Brenda, Philip and Tom whose healing touched my spirit and gave me hope, and to Clive Fowle and the healing group at Acocks Green Methodist Church.

to the Bach Centre for their gentle system of healing.

to Sara for the speed and efficiency of her typing and the spirit in which she carried it out.

to Teresa for working with me on the idea for the jacket and for the final art work.

COPYRIGHT
ACKNOWLEDGEMENTS

Grateful acknowledgement is made for permission to reprint a short extract from *What's Really Going On Here* by Susie Orbach, published by Virago Press. A short extract from *Hunger Strike* by Susie Orbach, published by Faber & Faber Ltd. Reprinted by kind permission of A.P. Watt Ltd. on behalf of Susie Orbach. Two phrases from 'Four Quartets' by T.S. Eliot, published by Faber & Faber Ltd. Two phrases from *A Leg To Stand On* by Oliver Sacks published by Picador, reprinted by kind permission of Oliver Sacks, c/o Rogers, Coleridge and White Ltd., 20, Powis Mews, London W11 1JN, in association with International Creative Management, 40 West 57th Street, New York, NY 10019, U.S.A. 'For Hope,' from *Prayers for Hope and Healing* by William Barclay, Fount Books, Harper Collins Publishers Ltd. Permission applied for, to quote from *I'm Alive* by Jackson Browne and *New Morning* by Bob Dylan.

FOREWORD

It is a privilege to introduce this book by Vivienne Martin, a record of her own experience, which represents so well the courage, doubts and fears of people facing possible death or severe disability from advancing brain tumours or other intracranial disorders. She portrays the dreadful realisation of illness and its feared consequences for patient, family and friends, the steps of enquiry including medical consultations and investigations leading inexorably to surgery deep within the brain, and the experience of being in hospital before and after brain surgery.

As a neurosurgeon I appreciate this perceptive view of the patient's life in a hospital ward, struggling to stay an individual within the restrictions and daily routine, but incorporated within the ward's close-knit community, appreciating the needs and suffering of others, and finding companionship and comfort from hospital visitors, fellow patients, nurses and other hospital staff such as radiographers and encephalographers. Doctors and their visits are closely observed: it is always salutary to see one's practice through the eyes of others. Occasionally Mrs Martin's experience has been singular. For example in her abiding distress concerning the metal stereotactic frame and in her dramatic account of its fixation to her head she differs from the vast majority of patients for whom this experience is uneventful and readily tolerated. However, such idiosyncrasy enlivens the overall record.

Mrs Martin was treated in the Midland Centre for Neurosurgery and Neurology, a specialist hospital in Smethwick located in the North West of Birmingham, which was closed in January 1996 as part of National Health Service reorganization. Very many will join her in regretting the closure of this fine centre and in saluting its nurses and paramedical staff for their skill, kindness and devotion to their patients. In the same breath I salute Vivienne Martin, a woman of admirable courage and determination, whose experience in hospital illuminates our understanding of those facing the perils of brain surgery.

C H A Meyer FRACS
Birmingham
November 1996

PRELUDE

It was a fine sunny afternoon in early September with just a sniff of autumn in the air; a hint of dying leaves and summer's end. The park was teeming with family groups out to enjoy the sunshine, to hold onto the summer, before autumn's inevitable changes. The trees were heavy with leaves. The small lake glistened in the bright sun. Our children were running around in the play area, excitedly shouting and clambering, or claiming space for themselves on the slide or the swings. We were just another family group, a traditional nuclear set-up with comfortable lives, engaging in predictable and pleasant post-Sunday-lunch activity. As I watched my children play, I was gripped by a great fear, an enormous sense of foreboding. It was a feeling that I would not have dared to express, could not have expressed, to anyone. I looked at my children and I felt 'I might not see them here again'. I wanted to get away from that park as if it was the very cause of my panic, as if, by leaving the place, the fear would loosen its grip, then fade away. It seemed an irrational feeling, a ridiculous touch of melodrama on a safe sunny afternoon. I felt that if I left the park I would return to security and certainty. I would be able to bind up this foreboding with routine and normality, to cover this raw nerve with activity and with the myths we use to make sense of our everyday lives.

We returned to my mother-in-law's house, where we were staying. Then, later that day, we left and headed back to Birmingham, back home and back to the start of another week, another school term, and, for me, back to wait for an appointment with a neurologist to investigate the strange symptoms I had been experiencing for some weeks.

1

PART ONE

July – 5 October 1993

DEVASTATION

In late July we returned from a holiday in Italy, where we had spent two weeks with some friends, staying in an apartment belonging to a colleague of my husband, Tony. It had been an enjoyable holiday with good food and wine, and lots of opportunities to practise the Italian I had been learning for a year. The happiest days had been spent swimming in deep river pools with the children and an inflatable shark and crocodile. We arrived home on Tuesday 27 July, exhausted but happy to be back. The next day, the friends we had been with were moving house, so we went to help them pack.

On Thursday I woke up, still spent and exhausted, a feeling I had experienced since early June. I had worked that term, part-time, as a counsellor both at a local college, and for Cruse, the bereavement care agency. I had also done some teaching for the local authority tuition service. Although my total number of working hours was not high, I had felt quite drained and far more tired than my work could explain. The holiday, while welcome, had been tiring in its own way, and I was glad it was over and I could unwind properly. Later that day, a strange tingling feeling developed and spread from the left side of my mouth. It was there the next day and I still felt unaccountably tired. During the weekend it spread to the fingers of my left hand, and I made an appointment to see my GP. I was puzzled, but initially, not unduly alarmed. My doctor suggested I wait for two weeks, then return to see him if necessary.

There was no change in that period. I was given a blood test and told, once more, to return a fortnight later. The tingling continued, and while I was a little concerned, I still expected the feeling to go, and

5

tried to carry on as normal. I went to see U2 twice, at Wembley and Leeds. I also had a successful interview for some work teaching on a counselling course at one of the local adult education centres. But through all these activities the strange sensation continued. At the end of August we went to visit my father in Durham, and to spend a few days on Lindisfarne, the beautiful Holy Island joined at low tide to the Northumberland coast by a causeway. It is a place we find restorative, almost spiritual, and we visit it whenever we can.

The next time I saw my GP, he decided to refer me to a neurologist. I was rather alarmed at this, but glad things were being followed up. I had some idea in my mind that the condition was viral, would take its course and that, somehow by the end of the summer holidays, it would have gone. As I waited for an appointment date, and as the tingling continued down my left side, I became more worried. I would go to sleep at night, vainly imagining that I would wake up the next morning to find everything was normal. But each morning, the feeling was there, and as I came to consciousness, a sense of despondency rose in me.

I received a hospital appointment for October, but as the tingling grew stronger, I became more anxious. I returned to my GP. By now, in the back of my mind, was the vague fear that this could be a brain tumour, and I expressed this fear to Dr Gabriel. I was not sure whether or not it was a realistic possibility, as I had no understanding of the nature of my symptoms, but voicing this distant fear would, I felt, in some way rule it out. Dr Gabriel could see I was becoming increasingly anxious and managed to get me an earlier appointment in September.

I carried on as normal. It was during this period that we spent the weekend at the home of my mother-in-law in Billericay. Then Tony returned to the college where he works as an English lecturer, my son returned to school and my daughter started her first term at nursery. I enrolled for another term of Italian lessons, practised playing my saxophone and prepared for the new course I would be teaching.

A few months earlier, I had met Bernie, whose children also attended our local primary school. This was a new friendship but one I knew was important. Although I had not known her for long, I asked her if she would come with me to see Dr Anderson, the consultant neurologist to whom I had been referred. I knew she was the right person.

In mid-September, Bernie and I went to see Dr Anderson. I had heard good things about him and that meeting confirmed them. We were shown into the room to be greeted by a big Scottish man with a grey beard. I described my symptoms to him, and after he had examined me, checking on my sense of touch and my reflexes, I asked him what the cause might be.

'Well, what do you think it could be?' he asked in a deep warm voice.

This was a wise man. He was not going to create anxieties, but he would listen and respond to them.

'I wondered if it might be a viral or bacterial illness, or maybe a stroke. But my main fear is that it's a brain tumour.'

He said it was not bacterial, but that it could be one of the others. 'We'll need to have you in for tests.' He said I would need a brain scan initially and perhaps further tests such as a lumbar puncture. I told him that whatever it was, I wanted to know everything. My mother had died from ovarian cancer seven years previously, and for me the whole experience had been made more difficult by the seeming impossibility of finding out information. At the time, it had felt like a conspiracy to keep everything hidden. I was determined that this was not going to happen to me, and I felt a strong need to make this clear. As we left, I asked, 'If this is a brain tumour, could it be malignant?'

He said it could, but the first step was to do the tests. It was too soon to say any more.

Bernie and I left Dr Anderson and then went for coffee. As we sat, we talked over the appointment. In her warm and supportive way, Bernie enabled me to clarify what I had been told. My first impression of Dr Anderson was of someone I could trust. He was honest, direct and cautious. When I had asked him questions and named my fear, he had answered me truthfully. He had known I wanted a straight answer and he had given me one. I felt safe with him.

About a week later, a letter arrived from the Midland Centre for Neurosurgery and Neurology to inform me that I would be admitted for tests on 27 September. The arrival of that simple letter changed the way I felt. Up till then, I had been trying to deal with fears, but abstract ones, ideas of fears. When I saw the words 'Will you please attend this hospital for admission', it felt different. This was real; I knew then that it was no dream. I was facing a situation that was completely new to me. The prospect of a brain scan was daunting. While I knew the procedure itself was not frightening, the implications of it were potentially very serious indeed.

The day before my admission was my daughter's fourth birthday. We went, as planned, to the local safari park, a place she loves. She adores animals and plans to go to China, when she grows up, to conserve pandas. I felt separate from my children that day. As they shrieked with delight at the tiger cubs, and the monkeys trying to wrench away our windscreen wipers, I observed them as if from afar. I was inhabiting another world. Dazed and hazy, I was elsewhere; my apprehension about the next day removing me from the present.

Monday 27 September 1993

We left for the hospital that morning, skirting the city, just another car at the tail-end of the rush hour. Earlier, Tony had taken Stevie to school and Josie to nursery. A quiet undramatic goodbye, tinged, for us all, with sadness and, for me, anticipation. Just a brief separation. A few days at most. I knew the children would be well looked after. My mother-in-law had come to stay with us, to help out while I was in hospital. She is a good, kind person: someone who can give solid support without being intrusive. The children knew that with her, they were loved and cared for. But it was bewildering for them to see me go off and difficult for them to fully understand why I was going into hospital. They knew about the strange tingling and that I was going in so that the doctors could find out more about it, but I did not know in what way they made sense of this, or what hospital actually meant to them. They were both sufficiently intuitive and perceptive to realise that this was not a routine matter.

My previous experience of hospital had been for the births of my children. On each occasion I was fearful, frightened of what was to come. Each birth was difficult, but exciting and glorious in its outcome. I had never known such love as that which I felt for my babies: my son, so tiny and vulnerable with his wise and worried face, my daughter, so alert and so beautiful, with a look of bright-eyed

8

optimism. I would do anything for them. My love for them was at the very centre of my being and to be separated from them under such circumstances was hard. But still, it was just for a few days. They would find out what was wrong with me. The virus would take its course, or they would give me some drugs to cure it. Soon everything would be back to normal. The children would be happy at school. I would be back at work. I would play my saxophone and learn Italian. Everything would be fine. Nothing would change.

We arrived at the hospital, a modest structure, surrounded by the symbols of ordinary lives: mundane semi-detached houses, allotments, a school, a few tower blocks on the skyline. An undramatic building amidst the urban spawl of the West Midlands.

The main entrance, an impressive façade, with 'Midland Centre for Neurosurgery and Neurology' in large letters on the wall, fronted a new reception area and lecture theatre. We were directed to Ward D, along several corridors, taking several turns until I lost my bearings. We passed through double doors at the end of a long corridor and entered the ward, where a blanket of heat enclosed me. It was a long, narrow ward with a series of two-bedded bays on the left and a row of windows on the right, against which were arranged vinyl-covered armchairs, some inhabited by men in pyjamas and dressing gowns. At intervals, there were tables covered with vases of flowers and magazines. Halfway down was an office where I saw a nurse and the ward clerk. Nervously, I knocked and tentatively introduced myself, producing my admission letter. It reminded me of arriving at college for the first time, fresh from A levels and summer holidays. A new experience. New people. A sense of nervous anticipation. A bag packed with necessities: pyjamas, towel, toiletries; with the vital links with home: photographs, Walkman, tapes; and with the diversions: a film magazine with an article on Daniel Day-Lewis, and my Italian course. Kathleen, the nurse, escorted us further down the corridor into the women's section of the ward and led us to Bay 12, the last of the two-bedded areas. She left us to unpack while she went off to get the forms for admission. I sat on the unoccupied bed in the small stuffy room with its high windows, while Tony unpacked my bag and put my things in the locker. There was a sense of stillness and of quiet and efficient activity behind the scenes.

9

Kathleen returned with the admission forms and filled in basic details, as well as a brief outline of my condition and my previous medical history. I had entered this ward as an outsider, walked past people obviously identifiable as patients. I felt I was not one of them, this group of people strung out along the corridor, some alone in armchairs or lying in bed, a few in twos quietly chatting, the occasional figure shuffling up or down the corridor; I was part of the outside world.

Kathleen completed the form and wrote at the bottom, 'Self-caring on admission'. What an ominous phase. I wondered what it would say when I left: 'Unable to care for herself on discharge'? Then she fastened a plastic identity tag containing my name and hospital number around my wrist, and suggested I change into my pyjamas to await the doctor who would examine me.

And so I became a patient; I donned my comforting winceyette pyjamas, put on my slippers and shuffled out of the room to the vacant armchair opposite. The woman in the next chair introduced herself; she was the occupant of the other bed. Still in her clothes, a smart white shirt, a red cardigan and pleated skirt, Judy was outgoing and friendly. With the familiarity that can sometimes occur when stressful and unfamiliar circumstances bring strangers together, we were easily exchanging information about our conditions. We were both new arrivals and had been admitted for tests to determine the nature of numbness and strange tinglings.

Soon after, the doctor arrived, a tall blond young man with a warm and gentle manner. He did a thorough examination, checking on my sense of touch, reflexes, sensitivity to light, strength and heartbeat. I asked him about the cause of my symptoms. I did not expect him to speculate, but I felt it was worth a try. He said it was not possible to say at this stage. I would have a CT scan that afternoon, and on the basis of the result, a decision would be made on further tests.

Tony had left to call in at work, and, since it was lunchtime, Judy and I, both now dressed as patients, made our way to the day room for our meal. There, we joined the others and became submerged in the group. I felt as though we were passive recipients of the meal, part of an amorphous mass of patients, although this was not, in fact, the case. The staff related to each of us with kindness and good humour as individual members of a group. Yet I did not like this room. I felt

10

ill at ease and was relieved when lunch was over. I had no appetite anyway and was glad to escape.

Back in the corridor, four of us chatted. This was different. There was a warmth, a commonality, and as we shared our medical details and, by implication, our fears, my feelings of anonymity and isolation faded. We knew what it was like to be patients, each of us in our own unique situation, yet having something in common with the others. Emma, a retired teacher, was recovering from an operation to remove a benign tumour from her spine. Sue had injured her spine in a fall. Judy had numbness and tinglings and I felt as if my body was in two halves, one side tingling, the other unaffected. There was an ease and a warmth in our conversation and an immediate mutual support. This was all implicit. There was no need to speak of it. It was around us and between us; a shared understanding of uncertainties and anxieties.

A woman in white entered the ward. She went to the office and then came down to me. She was a radiographer and had come to take me for a CT scan. We exchanged pleasantries, and she briefly explained what it would involve, as we walked down to the scanner room. Inside was another radiographer and the CT scanner – a black-covered table leading into a deep, white archway, housing the machine. The two radiographers, Jean and Pauline, had a comforting almost maternal presence. They helped me onto the table where I lay flat on my back as they gently positioned my head.

'Now we're going to move you into the scanner. Nothing to touch you. Nothing to hurt you.' They went into the adjoining room to operate the scanner and look at the screens. The table slid smoothly into the white hole. It was light and spacious in there. Not claustrophobic, as I had expected. All I had to do was lie still. Then, starting at the top of my head, X-ray slices were taken of my brain – like taking the top off a boiled egg and slicing across at millimetre intervals. This took some time and every so often the table would move fractionally. I lay perfectly still. I did not dare swallow, or scratch my nose. All I could do, as I lay there, was to wonder what they could see on the screen as each time a light went over my head from left to right and back again. Then I heard the door open and they told me it was all done. The table slid out of the scanner and they helped me down.

11

'That was the first half of your scan. We just managed to slot you in between outpatients' appointments. We sometimes do that with ward patients. We'll do the second half tomorrow.' She seemed to be going to great lengths not to alarm me. I felt just a little uneasy.

Then, holding my arm in the armlock nurses use to support patients who are ill or unsteady, Jean took me back to the ward. She did this with great warmth and concern. Both radiographers had been quite lovely as I came out of the scanner. There was not just kindness, but comfort and support in their presence, in their whole demeanour.

I rejoined Judy, Sue and Emma, who took me back into the group again and asked me how it had gone. I knew I would not know the results until the next day. The radiologists and Dr Anderson, my consultant, would look at the pictures and then I would be told the results.

The rest of the day was quiet and uneventful. I wrote notes to the children, drew a picture of a panda for Josie and chatted to Judy. Tony came in that evening. The children were fine. His mum was doing a wonderful job and keeping things calm and secure for them.

Tuesday 28 September

Judy and I woke early and resumed chatting. In less than 24 hours we had ceased to be strangers. There was an ease in our friendship which had developed remarkably quickly and was not just because we were both patients.

I decided to get dressed that morning. I did not want to stay in pyjamas and dressing gown. I was not ill. I needed to feel like myself, and not a shuffling figure in nightclothes. Although this was in a sense an act of defiance, it was an inner one and not directed at the staff, who were friendly and relaxed and would not see my being dressed as an issue. It was simply a small act of self-assertion and self-expression at a time when I needed to hold onto a sense of myself.

There was an atmosphere of peace and quiet activity on the ward. The staff were engaged in calm and efficient work. Patients held low-voiced conversations muffled by the still warmth coming from every radiator. The occasional figure would pass our room.

Around ten o'clock, the haematology technician arrived. Judy had warned me the 'blood lady' would probably come for me. Apparently

I had missed her yesterday when I was admitted. We greeted her with an ironic delight that left her a little bemused. We told her she was the highlight of our morning, although we knew there was coffee-time and the WRVS trolley to look forward to. Such were the events of the ward: calm monotony punctuated by short visits, each one absurdly appreciated in its own way.

With the skill and confidence of experience, the 'blood lady' found my vein and with barely a scratch inserted the needle and withdrew several phials of blood. This, she told me, was 'just routine', although I could not quite see what they planned to do with it all!

The morning continued, not unpleasantly: coffee, a short wander up the ward, desultory conversation, trips to the bathroom, a browse through each other's magazines.

A woman in white entered the ward. We all looked up. Whenever anyone in uniform came through the doors, patients would glance up, wondering, 'Have they come for me? Perhaps this came from a sense or even hope of monotony being disturbed or perhaps it was from anxious expectation.

It was Jean, the radiographer from yesterday; it was me she had come to see.

'Hello, Viv. I've come to take you down for the second part of your scan. We only had time to do the first part yesterday. We often squeeze in scans for ward patients where we can.' She seemed to feel the need to repeat yesterday's explanation. 'The scan will be just like yesterday but a doctor will inject some dye into your hand.' I accompanied her almost casually to the scanner.

Pauline, the other radiographer, was there again. A doctor did the contrast injection in my hand, and then I was positioned on the table.

'We are going to move you into the scanner now, Viv. Nothing to touch you, Nothing to hurt you.'

Once again, I lay still as the light went back and forth over my head. An infinitesimal shift of the table, then the light would pass over me again, recording another thin slice of my brain. I did not scratch my nose, twitch or tilt my chin, and I tried not to breathe too hard.

The scan was over and Jean took me back to the ward; her manner once again was kind and supportive. I would see Dr Anderson that afternoon when he did his ward round, and then all would be revealed.

I lay on my bed and wondered how the children were. Then a doctor appeared in the doorway and introduced himself. He was Dr Tembo, Dr Anderson's registrar. He gave me a brief neurological check and asked me about my symptoms. I was a little puzzled as to why he had come. I had a vague sense that his presence was not just to check on my condition. He was pleasant and kind, but I felt there was more to the visit. I had sensed something too in the body language of the radiographers: a subtle shift in their friendliness and kindness to a deeper human concern, an unconscious change in the way they related to me.

Then, very clearly and directly, Dr Tembo said, 'The scan has shown there is a small swelling on the right side of your brain. It is very deep and we do not know whether it can be reached. We cannot be sure what it is – we'll do further tests. You may be referred to a surgeon, but the swelling could be too deep for a biopsy.'

I sat on the side of my bed, my strength draining from me, my head hanging, my arms and legs limp, trying to grasp this short statement. He had told me, in a straightforward and honest way, what the situation was. He had not skirted around the truth nor had he used euphemistic language.

He left me briefly alone to register his words and went off to find the ward sister to be with me. Molly soon appeared: a small blonde Irishwoman in a smart blue sister's uniform. She found me sitting there, tears just starting to fall. I felt a firm, warm arm round my shoulder. She led me away to find a cup of tea. Dazed, I followed her. Childlike, I did as I was told, grateful for her concern and control. I could not think for myself. Tears rolling now, fears blinding me, I trailed along, dimly aware of Judy and the others looking up as we passed.

With hot tea, in a paper cup, we returned to the room. Tasteless tea. The symbol of concern, of the need to comfort and to be comforted.

Judy came in and joined us and then I cried. I wept. I could find no words.

'Shall I go and ring your husband, Viv?' Molly asked. I knew he would be in at any time but I could not find the words to explain this. She repeated the question several times. Judy sat beside me, her arm round me, and I wept. Both she and Molly allowed me to do this, and also tried to rationalise my fears.

Molly locked her eyes onto mine and said, 'Now nothing is certain, Viv. We don't know what this means. Let's not jump to any conclusions.' Her intense voice gave me no choice but to hear her words.

Then Tony appeared and silently put his arm around me. He had just seen Dr Tembo in the office, and had been briefly put in the picture, although he had not had the chance to take anything in. Molly told him the same as she had told me, went off to get him some tea, and then left us alone.

We did not know what to do with ourselves. There is something about a shock of this nature which simultaneously drains away strength and yet produces energy. When I was first told that my mother had cancer, and that it was too advanced to remove or cure, I could not keep still. After the phone call at 10.30 at night, I could not sit down. I walked the streets. I even did the ironing. I packed our bags for the dash up to Durham the next day, my son's first birthday.

Briefly, we sat on the side of my bed. Tony in shock and silence. Me in shock and tears. And so restless. I could not sit still. We went for a walk. Up and down the car park. Again and again. Backwards and forwards. To and fro. The autumn sunshine, bright and bleak. I looked back at Ward D, this low unassuming building, deceptively housing such scenes of quiet drama, such stark moments of shock. Not knowing where else to pace, we sat in the car. Only the previous morning, I had sat in this seat on my way here. The old familiar car. It felt like home. It felt safe. Whereas that place: that place which contained the unknown, the unexpected and the shocking – I did not feel safe in there. I was a stranger in that strange place.

I looked to the horizon. I wanted to drive, to drive and drive. Away. Away from this place and all it contained. Away to somewhere safe. Away where I could shake off the traces of all I had been told. Away to my children. To scoop them up in my arms, and get away, as far away as possible. But there was no 'away'. There was nowhere to go. Wherever I went, I would take this with me. I could go nowhere but back inside the hospital. So, reluctantly, we made a start. We sat for a while in the autumn sunshine on the wooden benches just outside the corridor of Ward D, and then slowly dragged ourselves back in, to await Dr Anderson's ward round.

I sat on the side of the bed and, soon after, I heard Dr Anderson's deep tones resonate down the corridor. He came in, accompanied by

Dr Tembo and Michael, his SHO. There was a quiet, almost respectful seriousness about them all. In all his years of experience, Dr Anderson must have seen this kind of situation many times. Yet this was a man who would not have been dehumanised by such experiences; he was someone whose humanity would have been enlarged and deepened by his work and his relationships with his patients. There were no obvious, easy words but a depth of feeling that was implicit in his whole demeanour. His words themselves were straight and to the point. He repeated what Dr Tembo had said, and told me the swelling was about the size of a marble.

'Would you like to see the CT pictures of it?'

'No,' I said immediately, although I regretted this soon afterwards. It was as if I had thought the pictures were none of my business. I think at that early stage of shock and disbelief, I had not quite realised that they were indeed my business and that they did have something to do with me.

'What do you think the swelling might be?' I asked. 'Could it be a tumour?'

'Yes, it could. Or, it could be a kind of birthmark – something you were born with that has flared up. The difficulty is not what it is, but where it is. Because it's so deep, we may not be able to remove it or do a biopsy.'

He told me I would have an MRI scan on Thursday and possibly other tests, so they could find out more about it, and then they all left.

Tony stayed for a while and then went home to be there for the children at teatime. He would return later after putting Josie to bed.

Judy, my room-mate rejoined me, and she stayed with me. She listened, talked and supported me. This good person, whom I had only known since yesterday, stayed close to me both physically and emotionally. It seems that at the moments of our greatest need, the right person will be there at the right time. This was so true of Judy. Even with her own fears and uncertainties, she shared mine. She allowed me to express all I felt, and she kept me going.

Around six o'clock, she went to the day room to eat. I could not go. I did not feel like eating. I lay curled up in a foetal position on my bed. The deadly news was still seeping in through every pore and claiming me. Every cell in my body was changed by it. It infiltrated my whole being and my reality was forever transformed. What had seemed solid and real had been shown to be an illusion. Nothing was certain. Nothing could be counted on or taken for granted. And this new reality was central. It did not just hang over me, it was part of me. Literally and metaphorically, it was in my head. There was no escape. In the core of my brain and in the centre of my mind, I would carry it with me wherever I went. As I lay there, I put my hand up to my head as if to take hold of this thing in my brain, this unwanted presence, and pull it out. Over and over, I said aloud to myself, 'I don't want this. I don't want this.'

I was still lying there when a visitor arrived. Chris, an old friend, had come straight from work. Smartly dressed, in her deputy head's clothes, she had just called in before going home. She had not expected to find a crumpled, shocked heap on a bed.

'Hello, Viv. How are you?' Still in her teacher's voice.

'I've just had a shock.' I heard my own distant voice.

She sat beside me as I explained. She put her arms around me and we both wept. Like a mother, she held me and rocked me gently and together we cried. I have known Chris for a long time and she has a deep and genuine empathy. She can easily express her own feelings, and in sharing my shock and desolation, and expressing her own, she gave me what I needed. The right person at the right time.

Then Bernie arrived. Once again I broke the news to a good friend. She listened as I blurted out the words. Then, in her calm and deeply caring way, she asked me to explain it again. She listened to every word I said, and questioned me closely, and in doing so, helped me both to clarify what I had been told and to express my profound shock. I knew she was with me at a very deep level and that her support was absolute. Again, the right person at the right time.

Tony came in later, after putting Josie to bed. He was tired and drained from the shock, from the everyday evening-time routine with children, and from the several phone calls he had made to break the news to family and friends. We were both exhausted. Before he left, well after the bell signalling the end of visiting, I asked him to make a phone call when he got home.

When my mother's cancer was discovered, it appeared that she had only about three months to live. They did not remove the tumour, but decided to use chemotherapy to control it. A friend of the family had recently been to see a spiritual healer, and, as a result, the arthritis she

17

had had for years improved tremendously. My mum was put in touch with Philip, the healer. She knew she wanted to live and she was prepared to try anything. It was not initially a question of belief, but, perhaps, one of desperation. However, I think, when she met Philip, she knew intuitively that he could help. It was clear the cancer was going to kill her, it was already so advanced, but she simply wanted to live for as long as she could. She had just retired from teaching, and after all her years of work, she was determined to have some time; time to spend with my dad, with her children, and with her grandchildren. She went on to live for 18 months after the initial diagnosis. Her survival surpassed the expectations of the doctors and she took pride and pleasure in this. My mum had great determination and the spiritual healing made a difference. It gave her the strength to cope with the gruelling treatment and it gave her the extra time she so wanted.

I asked Tony to ring Philip that night, to tell him what had happened and to ask him to send out absent healing. To an extent, it was a request from desperation. I did not know what to do at that time, but I had a strong drive to 'do' something. I thought I had to fight. We hear so often of people with serious illness who fight it, so I felt I must do that. But I did not know how. I could not be passive, but I had no idea how to be active. There was a swelling in my head and I could not do a thing about it. It is difficult to get to grips with something so abstract. Something you cannot see, or touch, just an image on an X-ray picture. I did not know what to do, or where to turn, so, in asking Tony to ring Philip, I was asking for spiritual help. It was not something I thought about. It was simply the thing to do.

After Tony left, Judy rejoined me. I knew I would find it difficult to sleep that night; my mind, although drained, would not rest. When the night staff came round at about ten o'clock, I asked if I could have a sleeping tablet. This I took straight away. I wanted to switch off, just for a while.

Wednesday 29 September

I emerged from this respite at around 2 a.m., and as I came to con-sciousness the realisation of what was happening rose once again to the surface, engulfed me, and then pushed me down, deep into an abyss of despair and hopelessness. I felt a desperate need for Tony and the children; I wanted so much to be part of their lives and yet somewhere deep inside me, I knew I had to face the fact that I might die. I knew then that I was ultimately alone.

I lay for a while, unable to go back to sleep, my mind relentlessly churning. The tears were coming and I did not want to wake Judy. I could hear the low murmurings of the night staff down the corridor and so I got up and trailed down to them. They pulled up a chair for me, sat me down and made me some tea. I let out my fears and my tears and they listened. They both accepted my feelings and rationalised them. They tried to make me see all was not lost. Then we talked about the prospective closure of the hospital and I briefly escaped into the realm of politics. At about 5 a.m. I returned to bed and dozed. Then Judy woke up, and we talked. She had the humanity and the courage to share my pain. She did not fear it nor shy away from it. By chance, she was sharing a room with me, and she accepted me and all my situation brought with it.

'Stay with your feelings, Viv. Accept them. Don't fight them. Just go with them.'

It was such good advice. I knew there was no running away from my situation. I knew I had to face it, and Judy, with her warm, firm tones, encouraged, maybe even 'gave me permission' to do that. I did not have to fight these feelings, nor push them to one side and deny them. I could only deal with this great sadness by accepting it.

That morning passed slowly. I sat on the sidelines and watched it go by. At some point, Michael, the SHO came onto the ward. I needed to ask more questions; I had been too stunned to ask many the previous day. He sat down with me and patiently and gently went over what Dr Anderson had told me yesterday. I heard the word 'stereotactic'. In the middle of the night the nurses had told me of a metal frame that was used for some brain surgery, including biopsy, and also for radiotherapy. He also briefly mentioned this frame.

At lunch time, I followed Judy down to the day room. I did not want to be there, but then I did not know where I wanted to be. Mechanically, I ate. I tried to chew my food. Then a woman came through the door carrying a big bouquet of flowers. She asked the nurses for me by name so I got up and went over to her. She introduced herself as one of my husband's colleagues. The college he works in is just a mile away from the hospital and the flowers were from her and the other lecturers in his staffroom. I could barely speak. I was moved that these people, some of whom I had never even met, had cared so much, and that she, Angela, had shown the compassion and courage to come into this place and give flowers to me. We walked down to my bed, and I thanked her. There was an honesty in her presence which meant so much to me. She worried that she had upset me by coming in. But she had not. It seems to me that you cannot upset someone by showing you care. The pain is there already; to allow its expression is beneficial and to be able to share deep feeling can only give strength. And this unknown woman had given me that.

Judy returned from lunch, went off to appropriate some vases, and then helped me to cut and arrange the beautiful pink flowers. It was good to immerse myself in this simple, companionable task. Judy had a way of keeping me moving while at the same time accepting my sorrow.

Soon after, a friend came in to see me. I had got to know her when our children were young, and while it was not a deep friendship, we had got on well with each other. As Suzanne approached, I could see she was distraught and barely able to speak. This was quite unexpected: Suzanne is an extremely kind person, but like many of us, her emotional life is kept firmly under control. Organisation and order are paramount in her life, and strong feelings are to be neatly and firmly packed away. She does not seem to find it easy to put her feelings into words, and that such powerful emotions had escaped had alarmed her. To lose control in this way was deeply frightening for her. She needed comfort and reassurance, and while she felt the need to apologise to me for being so upset, I felt there was no need. It had touched me that she felt so strongly that unaccustomed emotions had emerged, and it meant a lot to me to be able to give support to someone. I had received so much love and support over the previous two days, and I was glad to be given the opportunity to offer some.

I think it is likely the occasion had given me a sense of power and, in a situation where I was essentially powerless, I had subconsciously grasped the opportunity to take some control. I feel that many actions we take, however altruistic they may appear, have mixed motives, and I am sure that this occasion was no exception. It felt good to take the initiative and not to be at the mercy of my own overwhelming feelings.

20

So for a while we sat together and I held her hand, and after a while, she left.

That afternoon, Tony brought the children and Doris, his mother, over to see me. It was a fine, sunny afternoon and the staff were happy for me to go out with them all to the local park. It was the first time I would see my children after the shocking news of the day before. Tony came onto the ward to collect me and we joined the children and Doris, who were waiting in the car. The children were sitting there, bursting with energy and excitement, but with a wariness, a puzzlement on their faces. It was hard for them to see me emerge from this unfamiliar place. We all squeezed into the car and set off for the park, just a few minutes away. When we arrived, the children raced over to the slide, followed by Tony. As I stood with Doris, she put her warm, solid arm round me. I felt her strong, loving support.

'I just can't believe it.'

'I know. It's just not real. I can't believe it.'

'It's so unfair.'

'Yeah I know. It's just not fair.'

'I know. It's not real. I can't believe it.'

Round and round we went. What else was there to say? I looked at the children on the slide, Josie charging around and throwing herself into the fun with all her energy and enthusiasm, Stevie occasionally glancing back at me and his nanny. There was a frenetic quality and an anxiety in their play; at their own intuitive level they sensed something was wrong.

As I watched the children on the slide, it was as if I was watching through glass, as if I was already separated from them. I was picturing my children playing in a park; children without a mother, my children without me. If I were to die, it would change the course of their lives. They needed me. I wanted to be part of their lives. I could not bear to be deprived of that. And I stood there, so powerless. What could I do? How could I do anything? I did not know if anyone could do anything. All I knew, as I looked at my children, was that I wanted to live. Everything else in my life meant nothing. I simply wanted to live. I loved them and I wanted to be with them. Nothing else mattered.

We returned to the hospital and the children came into the ward. They were pleased to see mummy's bed, and when they met Judy, glad that mum had made a friend. But it was difficult for them to see

21

me in that strange place where I did not belong. There was an awkwardness and a bewilderment in their faces, and a kind of distance between us. For them, I belonged at home, as part of their lives, and by being in hospital I had somehow separated myself from them, and we were not able to enter into each other's experience. To play games, to climb on my bed, even to hug me was difficult for them. While I was in hospital, I was a stranger to them, and we did not know how to relate to each other. They could not bear to leave me but it was hard for them to stay. I could not bear to be parted from them, but I felt a kind of relief when they went.

Soon after, around teatime, two friends came in to see me, once again teachers, once again straight from work. They hugged me, and we sat and talked. Then it was time for me to go down to the day room for tea, so I left them briefly for about ten minutes. As I walked back up to my room afterwards, I wondered what I would find. Treas and Ange are known, amongst other things, for their sense of fun and their ability to turn any situation into an escapade which will later be turned into a funny story. As I returned to my room, I expected to find them playing some prank. And yet, there they were, sitting on my bed, quietly talking. I was amazed. I had been sure I would find Treas hiding under my bed and Ange going through the contents of my locker to find something to laugh at. I said this to them, and they both tried on my slippers, and we all practised the 'hospital shuffle'. While I knew that they cared for me, I feared that they would be uncomfortable with a show of emotion, and might see an expression of despair as a resignation to it. So, in helping to turn the situation into a game, in colluding with them, I was unconsciously seeking their approval. The effect of this was to give them a way of avoiding discomfort and at the same time to restore some degree of control to myself, at least over the way in which I was dealing with this. It was good for me to be able to see some humour in my situation, to indulge in some self-mockery and be silly. They allowed me, for the first time in those two grim days, to find that I still had some humour inside me and to express my feelings in that way.

After Treas and Ange left, I sat with Sue, one of the other patients. In a slightly hesitant, almost embarrassed voice, she said to me, 'You'll probably think I'm mad, Viv, but my sister's a healer, and she feels she can help you.'

'I don't think you're mad, Sue.' A wave of relief and disbelief swept over me. I told her about my mum, and that I had asked Tony to contact Philip, the healer in the North-East. Tony had told me earlier that he had rung Philip, but there had been no reply, so he had left a message on the answer machine. It seemed to me to be an amazing coincidence that Sue had approached me in this way, and that Brenda, her sister, had sensed that I would be open to spiritual healing and would not find anything weird or disturbing in being given this message.

When Brenda came in later to visit Sue, I went to meet her. My immediate impression was of a person of compassion. There was a solidity in her presence and, underlying her warm, down-to-earth manner, there was a kind of quiet authority. In her Black Country tones, she said, 'This is not what they think it is, Viv. Your time has not come. You will see your children married.' Brenda was making no claims in the way she said this. It was spoken in a low-key, almost understated way, but with a calm confidence. She knew, even without being told, precisely where the swelling was. At that stage I did not have a very clear idea of its location, but Brenda appeared to be able to sense exactly where it was. She was sending healing to all the patients, but for some reason, felt that she might be able to make a significant difference to my situation, and she had also intuitively known that I would be receptive.

When she said those words to me, it felt as if she had a deep knowledge, an access to truth, and in handing that truth over to me, she gave me a great, and a priceless gift: a gift which I simply accepted. I felt an immediate, almost a physical, lifting of a massive weight from my heart and mind. It was not a question of belief and I had no sense of clutching at straws. I would not have been able to do that. I had neither the strength nor the will. Even in that vulnerable state, I was capable of distinguishing between straws and a source of help that was substantial. I was not denying my situation by pretending it was not serious; I was not deceiving myself. I simply knew that this was a way through. I knew I had to face whatever lay ahead, but that when I had asked for help, in asking Tony to ring Philip, in some way I had been given help, given a source of strength and, above all, of hope. I am not religious, but I think I have within me an awareness of a spiritual dimension, a sense of 'otherness' and a

23

feeling that there is more to our lives than we can understand. And this gift of healing was something I did not need to rationalise, nor understand intellectually; I simply accepted it as it was given.

When Tony came in later, I told him what had happened. He told me he had sensed a transformation in me even as he approached. He too was aware of, and appreciated, the modest unsensational way we had been given this hope, and while he showed little reaction, it was clear to me that he accepted what Brenda had said without need for explanation or understanding.

Many friends visited that evening, and I drew on the love and concern that emanated from every one of them. One of the friends who visited was Margaret. Just a year before, she had undergone the shattering experience of cancer and the radical and gruelling treatment this had necessitated. She had faced all this with great courage and optimism. When she hugged me, I had a strong sense of her identification with me, that she shared with me an understanding of all this meant. She knew without words, and as clearly as anyone could know, what I was experiencing. Not only did she understand the initial shock and the sense of hopelessness and fear that immediately followed this, but she knew, too, the need and the inner drive to find a way of taking some degree of control, whatever that may mean, and the inner refusal to be a victim, a passive patient. She understood what it meant to me to be myself in the midst of all this, and the determination I felt to draw on any resource I could. Just before she left, Margaret gave me a copy of a poem from a book by William Barclay:

For Hope

O God,
It is very difficult to keep on hoping,
when nothing seems to be happening.
And it is even more difficult
when there seem to be more setbacks than progress.
Help me to have the hope
that nothing can put out.
After all, even on the darkest night,
no one ever doubts

that the morning will come again;
and in the hardest winter
no one ever doubts
that spring is never far behind.
Help me to think
of the skill you have given
to those whose task it is to heal,
and of the essential toughness
of this human body of mine.

This poem put into words what I needed. It is a prayer, and while I am not entirely comfortable with religious language, I felt the religious phrases of the poem contained an expression of a universal appeal for hope that transcended dogma and belief.

As Tony went home that night, some time after the end of visiting, I think we both felt that we had moved on a little from the shock and despair of the previous day. While I still felt fear and uncertainty, I also felt I had a glimmer of hope and a way to begin the attempt to handle this experience.

It had been an eventful day, packed with experience and feelings, a tough and demanding day, and I felt completely worn out. But my mind was still very active. I had had very little sleep the night before, and while I wanted and needed to sleep, I knew it would be difficult. I feared the night, the darkness it would bring, and it was a great relief when the staff came round with the drug trolley and I found that I had been prescribed two sleeping tablets. I had not wanted to ask, but I was very glad to receive them. I took them immediately and gratefully switched off and shut down for the night-time hours.

Thursday 30 September

Judy and I woke early to the welcoming sound of the tea trolley coming down the ward. As I surfaced from my night-time travels, the sense of shock was still present, but diminishing; the glimmer of hope was still there and the bleakness seemed a little less. I had had a good sleep, albeit a drug-induced one. Poor Judy, however, had been quite disturbed in the night. Apparently I had talked and shouted quite loudly and frequently in my sleep; even while my conscious mind was resting, my subconscious was doing its work.

We went down to the day room for breakfast, and one of the radiographers appeared. She had a questionnaire for me to complete in preparation for the MRI scan that morning. MRI scanning works through magnetism and it is necessary to ensure patients do not have any metal in or on their bodies. Fortunately I do not – although I was a little concerned about my mouthful of fillings. I had visions of teeth flying out, but apparently dental amalgam is safe enough.

Later that morning the radiographer came to take me for the scan. I had been told by other patients that, unlike the CT scan, an MRI felt quite claustrophobic and was noisy. As we left the ward and went along the cool passages and up the slope of the long main corridor, I felt quite nervous. I could hear a low, rumbling sound as we approached the doors leading to the back exit from the hospital. There, in the car park was a huge articulated lorry containing the mobile MRI scanner. We carefully mounted the steep metal staircase leading into the body of the lorry. Here were a radiologist and radiographers, a bank of buttons, dials and computer screens. To my left was a glass window and doorway into the scanner room. Just inside I could see a pair of legs on a table, the rest of the person enclosed by the sci-fi tube of the scanner. Buttons were pressed and the scanner table smoothly slid out to reveal a whole person. The radiographer went in and helped him to get off the table. As he emerged through the glass doorway, I scanned his face to see whether he had been through a traumatic ordeal. There were no obvious signs: he seemed a bit dazed, as I supposed anyone would who had spent half an hour lying inside a tube. There was even a trace of a smile. I decided the scan was probably not too bad. He was shown out of one door and down the steps as I was shown through the door on my left, into the high tech room which housed the scanner. I was helped onto the narrow padded table which led into the deep cavern of the machine. I lay on my back, and my head was carefully and precisely positioned. I was told that they would be able to speak to me and to see and hear me throughout the whole procedure. Then I was moved head first into the scanner, and enclosed by the dimly lit tunnel. I felt tiny and vulnerable: a small human figure confined in a huge futuristic machine. I closed my eyes almost immediately I was inside the tube. This was no place for the

26

claustrophobic. Through the background humming came a disembodied voice. 'Are you all right?'

'Yes. Fine, thanks.' Am I hell, I thought, but there was no other reply to give.

'We're starting your scan now.'

Buzz... Buzz... Buzz... Buzz.

Knock-knock... Knock-knock... Knock-knock.

Clank... Clank... Clank... Clank

The huge magnets came to life, all in syncopated time. For a machine at the forefront of technology it sounded remarkably 'Heath Robinson-like.' I wondered what the radiographers could see on their screens and what new information this scan would give Dr Anderson. I wanted to know everything about it. I wanted to be out there looking at the computerised images of the inside of my brain, to see inside my head and to know what it all meant. I wanted to hear everything the doctors said to each other as they discussed the contents of my head. I was so curious. And I was frightened. I thought of what Brenda had told me. I held on to that. I asked for healing and tried to radiate positive thoughts.

The noise stopped. The voice spoke.

'Are you all right?'

'Fine, thanks.'

'Another set of pictures now – about seven minutes.'

And so this went on. After about half an hour, the table moved out, and I emerged from the tunnel. The unknown was now familiar: if I ever needed another MRI scan, I would not be nervous in quite the same way.

I was taken back to the ward, where my partners in patienthood, Judy, Sue and Emma, were waiting to welcome me, and to hear how it had gone. It was very easy to share experiences with each other. There was no need for any of us to overdramatise or to underplay the procedures we went through; we could simply describe what happened and the experience would be accepted and empathised with. There was something quite restful and soothing about sitting in that small group in the corridor.

Lunch, however, was a more chaotic and surreal affair. The corridor down to the day room was inhabited by builders and lumps of wood which Sue, with her two sticks, somehow managed to negotiate.

The nurses were valiantly attempting to distribute lunch, and other medical staff were popping in and out. Sue got up to leave the room, and struggled to the door, only to find her exit blocked with planks of wood and workmen. She turned to a group of us and said, with a wry smile, 'It's like a madhouse in here,' and we all collapsed in hysterical laughter.

A sense of hysteria had been building up between Judy and me for days. We shared a similar sense of absurdity, and by Thursday the build-up of tension and emotion was such that we shrieked with laughter at the slightest provocation. Every so often, Judy would offer me a biscuit. The drugs she was on seemed to be making her ravenously hungry. I, on the other hand, had barely been able to eat for the last three days, and she had been quite concerned about me. Every time she devoured yet another biscuit, she would say to me, 'Fancy a Hob Nob?' and we would be off into a fit of giggles. When I told Judy about my MRI scan, I told her how I had been lying there, trying to think positive thoughts, but that every so often the image of one of the young doctors would surface in my mind. 'I hope the scanner didn't show what kind of brain activity was going on!' Once again we shrieked with laughter.

Every women's magazine we read contained articles on health: but we could take nothing seriously. As we turned a page and discovered yet another 'Women's A–Z of Health', we would collapse once again into a heap of hysteria. The irony of the articles was not lost on us as we lay there in our hospital beds. 'We weren't ill till we came in here,' we would often repeat to each other, in what may have been a subconscious attempt to blame the hospital for the predicament we were in.

The humour itself was, I think, a coping device. It was a means of releasing tension and emotion. In some ways it may have been an assertion of power in a situation where we felt essentially helpless: there was at times a cruel edge to our laughter. I think it was also an attempt to distance ourselves from our own situations: to stand back and indulge in some self-mockery was a way of protecting our vulnerable inner selves.

During that afternoon, Michael, the SHO, came in to give me the preliminary results of the scan. He said the picture had revealed two concentric circles showing evidence of bleeding and that the swelling appeared to be fairly self-contained. The next step would be a cerebral angiogram – this was an X-ray picture of the arterial layout of the right side of my brain. This would be arranged for the next day, Friday, or possibly the following Monday. This new information was apparently a hopeful sign. It was something else for me to assimilate, a tiny piece of jigsaw which I did not know quite where to place. But I was glad of it. I wanted to know as much as possible. As the doctors continued their search for more information, I felt a sense of movement, of no longer being quite so stuck. I knew that in his quest for a full picture of my condition, Dr Anderson would be absolutely thorough and tireless. I had had a niggling worry at the back of my mind for some time but had been too self conscious to voice it. Tentatively I tried out my question on Michael. 'Is it possible that this could have been caused by playing the saxophone – by the pressure inside my head, when I blow?'

Although I felt quite silly asking the question, Michael took it seriously. He thought it unlikely but said he would check with Dr Anderson, whom I was to see the next day. It was a relief to voice this fear, this sense that I might have been in some way responsible for my illness. And I was pleased to have my question taken seriously as I had known it would be.

Earlier that day, a woman who had been admitted the day before with a suspected brain tumour was taken down for surgery. The growth, which she had told us was the size of a golf ball, was affecting her memory. Betty was a lovely lady; gentle and honest in her vulnerability. When the theatre staff had come to collect her, a few of us waved her off and wished her well. I felt a sense of identification with her and found myself imagining what it would be like if I was ever taken down to theatre. I felt her fear, her uncertainty as to how she would be in a few hours' time. I wondered how I would be, if it were me, and particularly who I would be. What happens to our sense of self when the brain is invaded?

Later that afternoon, I was walking past one of the bays in the men's section of the ward and through the window I glimpsed one of the nurses shaving someone's head. I thought, 'That will be me, one day.' I realised it was wishful thinking and that I actually felt envy for these two people who were having brain surgery, these two people who had things which were accessible and possibly removable. I had the naïve

29

and selfish feeling that brain surgery was the simple way out, and that they were lucky to be undergoing such an operation.

Again that day I had many visitors. I received cards, gifts and flowers, and with every one there was love and good wishes; these were a genuine source of strength, something which I valued deeply. Again, I wrote notes and drew pictures for my children. This was a vital link between us. I had felt so separate from them the day before and in some ways I was preserving that distance. The preoccupation with my own condition, the identification with other patients, my locking into the hospital world, were ways of coping with this enforced separation. In finding something positive to draw from my situation, to value in it, such as the humour and camaraderie, I was protecting myself from the full horror of it.

After visiting had finished, Judy and I settled down to watch *Absolutely Fabulous*. The programme's hysterical edge ideally suited us at that time, although I suspect that our exaggerated shrieks of laughter did not suit the two men who had the misfortune to have been moved into the bay next to ours. I was dimly aware that we might be disturbing them, but not aware enough to tone it all down. They finally got some peace when the night staff did the drug round. I still feared the night approaching and was too wound up to sleep; so, once more with some relief, I took sleeping tablets. These enabled me to escape for a while, although again I disturbed Judy with my night-time shouts and ramblings.

Friday 1 October

We woke very early, some time before the tea trolley, and Judy and I carried on talking. In a week, a good friendship had developed and we had shared many aspects of our lives. However, 5.30 in the morning was perhaps a little early, and again we were disturbing the patients next door. The nurse on duty came down to see us and asked us to be quiet. So, like two naughty schoolgirls, suitably rebuked, we did as we were told, and, as soon as she had gone, stifled our giggles. Then we lay in silence to await the arrival of the tea.

One of the patients next door had undergone an angiogram the previous day and Judy had told him that I would be having one on

Monday and was nervous. 'Don't worry,' he said. 'It's a piece of cake. You'll be fine.' This was said with great kindness, and while it was said to reassure me, it was also spoken truthfully. It was as if he was saying with a grin, 'Look at me. Here I am. I've had one and I'm fine. You'll be fine too.' And these words were appreciated.

I saw him later sitting in an armchair in the men's section of the ward. He looked pale and miserable, so I sat down beside him. 'Are you okay?' I asked.

'I'm okay. It's just – I hate it in here so much.' And there was a panic in his voice, a sense of inexpressible fear, of feelings stifled by the oppressive atmosphere and the expectations of others. It seemed to me that the struggle to cope, to be seen to be coping with his situation, to be holding himself together for the benefit of those around him, and to preserve his self-esteem in the face of their expectations, was a huge burden for him. This was true, to an extent, of all of us, but perhaps the greater social and psychological pressures on men to preserve this façade put them under more strain than those of us who had the opportunities to openly and freely express our fears.

Tony came in just before lunchtime, and, soon, after, Dr Anderson, Dr Tembo and Michael came to see me. Dr Anderson's safe, solid presence seemed to fill the room.

'How was your MRI?' he asked kindly.

'Well, I could think of better ways to spend half an hour,' I retorted wryly.

He smiled at my weak attempt at humour and told me in more detail about the results of the scan. There was definite evidence that the swelling in my brain had been bleeding within itself. I asked him if this indicated any more clearly what it could be. He told me there were still two main possibilities. It could be some kind of tumour or it could be a kind of cyst or birthmark – something that had been sitting there to no ill effect for all of my life, but had now 'flared up'. At one point in my questions, I referred to the swelling as 'inaccessible'. Dr Anderson quickly corrected me on this, and more precisely described its location as 'difficult to access' rather than inaccessible. He asked me once again if I would like to see the pictures, and this time I said 'Yes'. I knew now that it was my business, and had everything to do with me. My initial shock had been replaced by a huge thirst for knowledge, and a need to understand as much as I possibly could

31

about what was going on in my head. Again, I think, this was a means of coping, of confronting my situation. I felt I could not begin to get to grips with this presence in my brain, and in my mind, unless I knew what I was trying to face.

So Dr Anderson held my scan pictures up to the window and I gazed upon the scene of my devastation, the radiological image of my shock. There it was, facing me, a clearly distinguishable circle, neatly self-contained, lying in the middle of my brain. Blatantly sitting there where it had no right to be. Yet it was part of me. I might have been born with it. As I looked upon this image of myself, I had no alternative but to accept it. I was it. The subject became the object.

Seeing those pictures was valuable for me. It made it clear to me that this was no bad dream, that this swelling was real and was actually present. The abstract was made concrete: on the right side of my brain, deep down, towards the centre, was a swelling of some sort, a 'lesion'. What it was could not be known for certain, what it would do was equally uncertain, and what, if anything, could be done about it was doubtful. Seeing the scan pictures made it all real to me, at the same time enabling me to step back and to look at the evidence with objectivity. The distance this afforded me was helpful, was a way of coping with the unimaginable.

Dr Anderson confirmed that I would have an angiogram on Monday, and then, to my delight, said that I could go home for the weekend. I self-consciously voiced my question about the saxophone. He thought it unlikely that I had caused the swelling in my brain to bleed, but thought it wise not to play it until the results of the angiogram were known.

I then asked, 'Could I have a gin and tonic?' meaning 'Would it be all right to have any alcohol?' while this was bleeding in my head.

He smiled and said, 'Yes, in moderation.' I did not actually intend to go off and get plastered, but I am sure it was reasonable to assume that I might consider it in the circumstances.

The doctors went off and Tony went over to college for an hour while I gathered together my belongings.

Judy too, was going home, although unlike me, she would not be returning. Once she was ready to leave, we said 'Goodbye' and exchanged addresses and telephone numbers. It seems to me that in such circumstances, addresses are sometimes exchanged as a means

32

of easing the difficulty or embarrassment of a goodbye to a relative stranger we have got to know briefly or intensely. There may be no real intention or likelihood of staying in contact but it is often more comfortable to act as if we will see someone again. I was sure, however, that Judy and I would keep in touch. The common bond which had developed between us was more than transitory and far from superficial.

Soon after Judy had gone, Michael arrived with a detailed explanation of the angiogram and a consent form for me to sign. Then I wandered into the bay next door, where a new patient had been admitted. She was a young woman in her early twenties. She lay in her bed, a soft toy in her arms, and she looked frightened and vulnerable. Tears were rolling down her cheeks. Her mother and sister appeared and told me she had multiple sclerosis and that it had affected her speech. Patricia watched and listened to this conversation, and nodded. Her sister explained that she felt self-conscious about her speech, and Patricia nodded again. They were warm, kind people, and did not seem to mind my intrusion. I felt welcomed by them and we chatted for a while.

When Tony returned we picked up my bags and hurriedly left the ward. Yet, as I went out through the main doors of the hospital, I felt a tremor of insecurity. I sat once again in the passenger seat of the car, where I had slumped in despair three days earlier, and we headed off, taking the route I had fantasised about in Tuesday's urgent need for flight. I wanted to go home, I wanted to be with Tony and the children at home, and yet to disengage from the hospital was difficult, knowing that I had to return at 8 a.m. on Monday. It was as if I did not dare let go of the place completely. Whatever survival strategies had enabled me to get through the last few days could not be allowed to crumble, not when I might need them in three days' time. I still had to motivate myself to return, and I think this may have been part of the reason why I befriended Patricia. Perhaps I wanted to be needed, and needed to find a role for myself, a purpose and justification for going back.

Half an hour later, we arrived home to find the reassuring figure of Doris, pot of tea at the ready, waiting to welcome us into the house. I wanted so much to see the children on their own ground and looked forward to them returning from nursery and school.

It felt unreal to be in the house again. Home seemed familiar yet so strange. I felt I did not quite belong there. It was as if the house was the property of other people, and of the woman I had been when I left at the beginning of the week. The person entering now was a dreamlike figure, dissociated from this home: an alien being with a strange formation in her brain, a being with an uncertain future. I felt as if I was no longer part of this place; it was known to me yet I was separate from it. I knew it from a different existence, one where life was safe and could be counted on. But this figure I had become could count on nothing. The only thing I could be sure of was that certainty is an illusion.

I sat down and waited for the children. I did not know what to do with myself. It was hard to sit and do nothing and yet activity for its own sake was empty and meaningless. I felt rather lost. I did not dare to feel too much at home. I could not allow myself to feel too secure and settled when I knew I had to go back to hospital. I felt restless and ill at ease. Then, to my relief and delight, Josie arrived home. She bounded in and leapt on me, then immediately demanded juice and something to eat. Like a whirlwind, she swept through the house, carrying everyone with her, then she settled, exhausted, panda tucked under her arm, and watched television for a while. Occasionally she would give me a suspicious glance, as if to say, 'What are you doing here? Are you staying? Can I trust you to stay?' She was delighted to see me but worried at the same time, and I think this was reciprocal. The pain of my love for her frightened me.

Later in the afternoon, Stevie returned from school, his gentle, sad face lighting up when he saw me. School had become the focus of many of his anxieties about me, and he immediately told me what an awful day he had had. His notes to me in hospital would often say, 'I love you mum, but I hate school.' But I failed to pick up just how strongly the two statements were connected. Stevie had never been unhappy at school, and I should have realised that what he was feeling about school was essentially a projection of his fears about me. But I was so locked up in my own world, I failed to recognise this and to help him address his fears.

Even though I felt separate and removed from all that went on around me, Friday evening seemed relaxed and pleasant. I was glad to sit and watch television with the children, and to play my part in

34

routine bedtime activities: to experience just a taste of normality in the midst of all that was extreme and extraordinary was a relief. I slept well that night – I had no sleeping tablets and no need for them. I was glad to be in my own bed.

On Saturday, my dad was to arrive for the weekend. My sister was also planning to visit. The news about me had shocked them very deeply. They had always identified me with my mother, and did so particularly after her death. While we did resemble one another in some aspects, there were many differences. I felt nervous about their visit. I knew that they would compare my situation to that of my mother. I feared that their feelings would overwhelm me and that they might find it difficult to differentiate between us. I felt I had to make it clear to both of them that what I was facing would be dealt with in my way, that I had no time for pretence and clichés. I would describe my situation as it was and face it as it was. So when they arrived on the Saturday morning, I hugged them and then spoke fairly brusquely and directly before either of them had time to speak.

'Right. This is the situation. There's a swelling in my brain. They are not sure yet what it is. It may be a tumour or a kind of birthmark. The problem is not just what it is, but where it is. It is probably too deep to remove and may be too deep for a biopsy. The test on Monday will give them more information, so we will know more then. Do you want some coffee?'

And so, in this cruel and blunt way, I defined my own position. When my mother was ill, information was kept from me. This time I was in control, and I did not want to play euphemistic games. And to their credit, they accepted my way of dealing with things. The opportunity to talk to my sister and the solid love I felt from my dad were a great help and comfort to me.

The remainder of the weekend passed in a relaxed but, for me, hazy sort of way. I felt remote and preoccupied. Although the prospect of the angiogram worried me, I was anxious to return to hospital and get on with it. I could not fully 'be' at home, knowing I had to go back. In addition there was still more to learn about my condition, and I was eager for this information. My fear had produced an enormous need for knowledge. And although I knew nothing could eliminate the fear – it was as if it was structural and could not be removed – any information I could gain would at least help me to know as fully as possible what I was facing.

I went to bed on Sunday night, full of nervous anticipation but prepared and ready to go back into hospital the next day.

Monday 4 October

I woke early on Monday morning and rinsed my mouth out with tea: I had been given strict instructions that from Sunday night it was to be 'nil by mouth'. Then I bid an anxious goodbye to the children and reminded them that I would come back home soon, probably in the next two or three days.

Once again, we made the early morning drive across the city, home behind, hospital in front. One week on, I was re-entering Ward D, but this time not as a new arrival; all the staff were familiar and so were most of the patients. The few that had remained for the weekend were having a peaceful and leisurely breakfast in the corridor and welcomed me back as we came down the ward.

Once again, I went into Bay 12 and we unpacked my bag. I was very conscious of Judy's absence. The place felt different without her; it seemed somehow more serious. I found it difficult to tune back into the atmosphere of the hospital after my break at home. The calm activity of the ward was at odds with the restless way I felt.

Tony went on to college and I chatted with the other patients for a while. I could not settle to read nor listen to music. The prospect of the angiogram loomed ahead. I felt, despite reassurances, that it could be an unpleasant procedure. I was given a theatre gown and paper hospital knickers to wear. I asked the staff if I would be given any form of pre-med, and, in my anxiety, repeated this question several times. I was given a sedative tablet and an injection in my leg. I think I had hounded the nurses so much and radiated so much fear that I had left them little alternative. However, the effect of these drugs was not to reduce my fear, but to make my body feel like lead and to give me a sense of powerlessness.

Soon after, the black trolley arrived to take me down to the X-ray department. I was loaded onto it, and taken speedily along the cool corridors, past towering shelves of files, round tight corners and into a gloomy room, heavy with machinery, where I was greeted by the radiographers. By this time, my fear was so great, every limb was shaking. I tried, but I could not keep my legs still. Yet these involuntary movements seemed to be the only ones I could make; I felt so heavy and helpless. I was moved from the trolley onto the X-ray table. Then the radiographers cut open the paper knickers and stuck on heart monitor pads. I felt quite embarrassed about my shaking legs, but I just could not keep them still. The radiologist then appeared and injected local anaesthetic into the right side of my groin, before inserting a catheter into the right femoral artery. I felt a deep pain as this went in. The radioactive dye was injected, a large black camera was brought over my head, and pictures were taken of the arteries on the right side of my brain. Hot impressions of these vascular pathways went through my head and then were gone.

The radiologist removed the catheter and applied pressure to the punctured artery. While he did this, the radiographers removed the heart monitor pads. Then I was gently and carefully lifted across onto my bed and wheeled back to the ward. The whole procedure seemed to be over with a speed and efficiency that almost made a mockery of my anxiety and my quivering legs. Once again, it was shown to me that fear of the unknown is far greater than fear of the known. It seemed to me to be unlikely that I would ever need another angiogram, but I knew if I did, I would not be afraid in the same way.

For the rest of that day, I lay dazed and apart from everyone. The bed that had been Judy's was empty. I was not allowed to sit up or move for 24 hours because of the punctured artery in my groin. The sedatives I had been given removed me from active communication with anyone. I felt very lonely and cut off, but I could do nothing about it. I would know the results of the angiogram the next day, but until then I had to lie flat and use bedpans. At one point, Dr Tembo and Michael called in to see me, but I was too dazed to talk to them. Patricia's mother came to see me and filled the room with her concern and her warm smile. By the evening, the drugs had worn off, and I was allowed to move around a little. I spent some time chatting with Sue and Emma, their gentleness and kindness comforting and soothing me, and I sat with Patricia and her mother. Once again, the contact with other patients, the implicit communication between us, broke through my isolation and gave meaning to being in the place.

Tuesday 5 October

I went in to see Patricia that morning. She seemed to be withdrawn and deeply unhappy. I sat and held her hand and we talked. We were quite comfortable with each other and while her speech difficulty limited what she could say, communication between us was easy and natural. I think she may have felt safe and comforted by my presence. I, in turn, was glad to fulfil my own need to support and to protect; a need which may have come from my own projected fears and vulnerability. Whatever the subconscious motives, it felt good to be able to give something.

Later that morning, I was moved into the four-bedded room next door. This was a welcome contrast to the dark, two-bedded bays with their high windows, huge radiators, and stuffy atmosphere.

The 'Wendy House', as it was affectionately known by staff and patients alike, was a bright and airy room, a modern extension to the ward. Sue had also been moved into this room, although I knew she would be going home later that day. We had already exchanged addresses and telephone numbers and I was sure we would keep in touch. I knew I would also stay in touch with Brenda, her sister.

Tony called in that morning, and soon after his arrival, Dr Anderson did his ward round. My angiogram had shown that the swelling in my brain was not arterial, was circumscribed and not extending into surrounding tissue. Apparently, many malignant brain tumours, although not all, are vascular, and so the results were hopeful. It was still not possible to know for certain what the swelling was, and the risks of biopsy at this stage far outweighed the risks of leaving it alone. Dr Anderson's feeling was to wait a few weeks, and then scan it again to see if there were any changes. He gave me this information in a way that lifted my hopes. As always, he clearly and truthfully described the situation. He answered all my questions in his straight and direct way. He raised no false hopes, but when he told me I could go home, he was enabling me to go with some hope, something which would help me through the waiting period. His advice was not to rush into a potentially risky biopsy, but to be patient. I felt completely safe and secure with him. He was not a doctor who took control away from a patient, and yet he was in control. I was able to feel that I was an active participant and not a passive victim. I knew I could trust Dr Anderson and that I could rely on his caution, his experience and his wisdom.

I was thrilled to know I could go home. My only reservation, as I repacked my bag, was that I would be leaving Patricia. I felt I was deserting her, as if I had extended the hand of friendship and was now taking it away. And yet, I was so excited to be going home properly, and with more hopeful news, that I could hardly get out of the hospital fast enough. Again, as I left that safe environment, I felt a tremor of insecurity, but I knew, when I arrived home, that I would 'be' at home and could relax there.

PART TWO

6 October 1993 – 6 February 1994

LIMBO

October 1993

It was good to be home. I felt that I was now able to put down a heavy weight. It seemed as if every muscle in my body had been straining to its maximum capacity in order to sustain the great load of the previous week. Every ounce of strength I possessed had gone into coping not only with the shock of the news I had been given, but also with the separation from my family and friends, and the adjustment to life in an institutional setting. It was a tremendous relief to let go of that weight. I had not been able to relax at home at the weekend, but this felt different. Family life could go on relatively normally and I could play my part in it.

The simple aspects of life at home were the easiest to appreciate: to sleep in my own bed, to make a cup of tea when I wanted one, to use my own bathroom, listen to the radio or watch television. To smell good fresh coffee. To turn music up loud and sing at the top of my voice. To walk in the garden. To swear loudly and with great venom. To cry in privacy when I wanted, and for as long as I needed, without having to stop when sympathy was offered.

Far more complex was the joy of being with the children. It was a relief to be part of their everyday lives but it was difficult. I felt very tired: whether this was a symptom of my condition or my shock, I do not know. While I wanted to be with them and play my usual role in their everyday lives, I felt I had no energy. I enjoyed the peace and

43

solitude when they were at nursery and school, but I missed them deeply. I was relieved and delighted when they came home. Yet at the same time I felt withdrawn and preoccupied. I found it difficult to engage in their world, to hear and to empathise with their concerns. For a while I was carried along by the joy of being at home and uplifted by Brenda's words and by the more helpful signs shown by the MRI and angiogram results. But, as the weeks passed, I still had to live with the knowledge, and the constant reminder from the tingling sensation, that there was a swelling deep within my brain. I feared it would bleed again and that it would grow. I felt insecure and alone. I wanted to ask questions. I wanted reassurance. But there was no one to ask, and, in any case, no reassurance that could be given. I felt helpless and had a need to act, to take some small degree of control.

Towards the end of October I wrote to the Bach Centre in Oxford. I had used Bach Flower Remedies on previous occasions, and while I did not have a clear understanding of them, I felt that they could help me. I was not looking for a miracle cure, but a way of living with and dealing with my situation. I knew complementary therapy such as the flower remedies and spiritual healing not only could provide me with a sense of taking some action for myself, but also would strengthen my resolve and determination. I knew the Bach Flower Remedies would help me to address the emotional aspects of my condition and find a way that was my own of coping with it. In my letter to the Bach Centre, I outlined my situation and then wrote,

> At present, I feel like I am walking an emotional tightrope of trying to be positive but also trying to face up to the uncertainties and the possibility this could be life-threatening. I am receiving spiritual healing which is a tremendous help and does give me a quiet confidence I will come through this. But at times the fears do take over and at times I feel quite exhausted from struggling with it. Being positive feels like a big responsibility; this is a good thing in the sense of giving me some control over my own health but is also daunting in the sense that if I'm not positive, will the swelling grow and take over.

By return of post they sent me two treatment bottles and a letter explaining which remedies were included and expressing concern and kindness. I immediately started taking the remedies, four drops four times a day. I knew they would help me to cope with the shock,

44

the fears and the tiredness, and would help me to continue the struggle.

Friends and family continued to give us support in a range of different ways. Our needs, both practical and emotional, were met by many people. Doris stayed on with us, and gave us her strong maternal love. We had many visitors, cards and letters, gifts and flowers. Good wishes came, not just from friends, but from friends of friends of friends. We felt that there was a network of love and strength available for us to link into and to draw on. Every single good wish, offer or gesture was appreciated and valued; each one helped. One day, during half-term week, I took the children out, and we returned to find a note and a chocolate cake waiting for us in the porch. This expression of concern from Wendy, the friend who made it, meant a lot to all of us, and was eagerly devoured. Bernie gave me strong and consistent emotional support; her understanding and acceptance of the complexity of my emotional responses was exceptional. Some friends offered us diversions and distractions. We had a night out at The Tower, a local dance hall, where I was able to lose myself in the sweet sounds of 1960s soul music and dance away my sadness and fear. It was during this evening that I started plans for my fortieth birthday party in January.

I kept in touch with Judy and Sue, my fellow patients. I regularly spoke to Brenda, the spiritual healer, on the phone, and on each occasion would feel uplifted and encouraged, not just by her words, but by an almost undefinable quality in her voice, and in the sense I had of her presence at the end of the line. I also spoke to Philip, the healer I knew in the North-East who was sending me absent healing.

Throughout this time, Tony was going to work as usual and helping to keep things as normal as possible for the children. He totally accepted my way of dealing with the experience; I felt completely supported.

A friend of ours lent me a book by an American surgeon, Bernie Siegel, in which he explores ways in which we can influence our own health. I found the book interesting and stimulating; in it he writes of the significance of the relationships between patients and doctors, and of the importance of expressing and understanding our reactions to illness.

One way of doing this, he suggests, is to draw a self-portrait, and to do this quickly and without conscious thought – the idea being that expressing oneself in this way will reveal unconscious attitudes to ourselves and our health and that often, at an unconscious level, we

45

may have a knowledge and an intuitive understanding of our illnesses. I immediately tried to do this before I had time to think consciously about it. My 'self-portrait' was a simple childlike drawing which, while it reflected my lack of artistic ability, nevertheless revealed to me some of my deeper attitudes towards my condition. One of the most striking relevations for me was that I had drawn the swelling in my brain as a large white circle; in fact, until I defined it later with a pink rim, the white wax-crayon circle could hardly be seen on the white paper. It seemed that I perceived the swelling as a barely visible part of me. I might have expected to see a dark, malevolent intruder: in the first few weeks after its discovery, I did think of the swelling in terms of an invader, and I did, on occasion, use battle imagery as a metaphor for my struggle. However, as the weeks passed, I increasingly saw it as a sad and unwanted presence. I felt almost sorry for it, as if through no fault of its own it was in the wrong place and had done the wrong thing. While my drawing showed that I perceived a large and dominating presence, I think the image I had of it was essentially benign. Perhaps in almost caring for it, and accepting it as part of me, I was finding a way of living with it at that time. There were occasions when, in bitterness or fear, I would refer to it as 'Quatermass', but overall, I came to feel a sense of concern and pity for this 'poor thing'. However, I had also drawn on the picture strong blue arrows driving the swelling out of my head. It seemed to be a case of, 'I'm sorry mate. It's not your fault you're in there, but I'm afraid you've got to go.'

My fears, however, were still present and were great. Even if the swelling was benign – and there was no physical evidence to prove this was the case – I had no means of knowing what it might do. A lot of the time I felt very frightened indeed: I knew my future was uncertain.

We had told the children that the tingling sensation was caused by a swelling in my brain, and that the doctors were not sure what it was, but would 'keep an eye on it' to see whether it changed or not. This was the only information we gave them at this stage; we wanted to tell them the truth even if it was a partial truth, and to speculate further would, we felt, have alarmed them unnecessarily. However, I think they sensed that my condition was indeed far more serious than I tried to make out, and I feel that I was not sufficiently aware of this at the time nor able to respond to it as sensitively as I should.

46

Josie used to return from nursery at lunchtime and was always very tired. She and I would sit together in an armchair, Josie tucked under my right arm, her panda, 'Babby', tucked under her arm. With a cup of juice in one hand, she would suck her lower lip and stroke Babby's fur as we sat and watched *Playbus* on television. I wanted to hold on to those moments for ever, and never let them go. I felt the deep pain of my love for her. I could hardly breathe as I felt her small, vulnerable presence beside me. I knew her need for me and my need for her. There were moments when we would look at each other and recognise the pain in each other's eyes. Without words, Josie seemed to sense my fear. But while I was dimly aware of this, I failed to consciously recognise it. I felt, as we sat together, how inextricably her beautiful young life was bound up with mine.

When I looked at my children, I knew that at the very core of my being lay my desire to live and my determination to live. I feel it is easy to assume we all want to live, but it seems to me that the desire to live is not so simple and cannot be taken for granted. Within many of us, perhaps all of us, there may exist an unconscious wish to accept illness or to contemplate death as an opportunity for respite or withdrawal from the complexities or ambiguities of living. I feared this possibility within me, this tiny subconscious suggestion that life was too big a struggle, that it was demanding and difficult. And as I recognised this possibility within myself and grew to fear it, I turned away consciously and deliberately and knew with absolute certainty the strength of my desire to live.

Around this time, I went with Bernie to see *The Piano*, a powerful and deeply affecting film. There is a scene towards the end when the main character falls from a boat into the ocean. Her ankle is caught by a loop of rope which is fastened around her piano. As the heavy instrument sinks and drags her down deeper and deeper towards her death, the camera focuses on her. We can see it is possible for her to unloop her foot and set herself free. But, for what seems like several minutes, she allows herself to be pulled down as she considers her decision. She could so easily allow herself to drown, to escape. We watch and wait to see what she will do. Then finally she unloops the rope from her ankle, and releases herself. She has chosen to live.

I was not conscious of this at the time but at some dim level of awareness, I felt a sense of identification with the character in this

47

scene. Although I was not in a situation where I had to make a simple choice between living or dying, somehow it was important for me to feel the strength of my desire to live, as well as recognise the possibility of a subconscious voice which might encourage me to relinquish the struggle. As I grew aware of and felt the fear and the lure of this seductive voice, as I heard it and said 'no' to it, I found somewhere within me a steel core of determination.

Co-existing with this resolve, and fuelling it, was the intensity of my love for my children, and the fear I would be ultimately separated from them: a fear so sharp that over the ensuing weeks I seemed to withdraw from them. I was not aware at the time that this was happening, but, over that period a distance started to develop between the children and me. It was a response to and a retreat from the painful fear of my illness and possible death. And it was mutual. There was an instinctive backing off on all sides, which may have been, at an unconscious level, a way of protecting our vulnerable inner selves from this immense fear that we would be separated by my death.

My own withdrawal was related, not only to my fear, but also to my preoccupation with my condition. I found it difficult to engage in aspects of everyday life. I felt as if I was in a separate, an 'other' world of my own. Aspects of my life which had previously seemed important now appeared superficial. My interests and hobbies were mere trimmings, trivial paraphernalia. Their meaning was peripheral and insubstantial. What had substance and meaning was my life itself. This was central.

November 1993

As the weeks passed since leaving hospital, I felt increasingly insecure. The tingling sensation seemed to be slightly stronger, although I could not be sure of this; my anxiety was such that I felt I might be imagining changes. I was not sure I could trust my own judgement and yet I felt I was responsible for monitoring my own symptoms. Every sensation, every headache, I experienced could, I felt, have been caused by the swelling growing or bleeding. As the time approached for my CT scan on 12 November I felt eager to go back to the hospital. I wanted objective evidence to show me what was

48

happening. I wanted to hand back to the doctors the responsibility for monitoring my condition. I was looking forward to seeing Dr Anderson again, and I needed to ask more questions. I felt there was a security in knowledge, whatever that knowledge might be. And if the scan gave Dr Anderson more information, I knew he would pass it on to me. I found not knowing what I was trying to deal with very difficult. In a sense, I still did not know what I was facing. Did I have years to live? Would I ever be fully well again? Or would I slip into a slow decline? Was I facing disability? Or death? Was I trying to come to terms with cancer? Or a lifetime of one-sided tingling? I felt I did not know what was happening. I wanted knowledge and certainty. And I hoped the scan would provide some answers.

I had worked on and written out a long list of questions. I was learning to be as precise as possible in my questioning. I knew Dr Anderson would answer me truthfully, but that to obtain the maximum information, I had to phrase my questions carefully and sometimes to ask the same questions in different ways.

Once again, I asked Bernie to accompany me to the hospital for the scan. Her intuition is as sharp as that of anyone I have ever known and she had a way of enabling me to express my feelings and fears, a deep understanding of my moods and my needs, and of my ways of coping with the experience. She also had the ability to listen with great intelligence and perception to the answers to my questions, and could enable me to sort out the important information and to clarify the central issues. Both Tony and I felt that in accompanying me to these appointments, she was helping not just me, but all of us.

On 12 November, Bernie picked me up and drove me to the hospital. It was strange to see the place again, both comforting and, at the same time, discomforting. We sat in the waiting room and I was soon taken through for the CT scan. Once again I lay on the narrow padded table, my head was carefully positioned and this time my body and arms were held in place by a strong fabric wrap.

'Moving you in now, Viv. Nothing to touch you. Nothing to hurt you.'

I lay still as the X-rays revealed the inside of my brain. Then the table was moved out and a doctor come in to give me a contrast injection in the crook of my arm. He joked light-heartedly with the radiographer. Then there was a sharp scratch as the needle went in. I was moved back into the scanner and I lay there still and silent. As the pencil of light moved backwards and forwards across my head, my mind moved to and fro. I thought the tingling had become stronger over the past few weeks, but only slightly. I decided I must be imagining the change: the stress of the situation was making my symptoms appear worse than they actually were. I felt, perhaps, I was taking the whole experience far too seriously, that I was indulging in it and being melodramatic in the way I felt. I thought other people would pull themselves together and get on with their lives. I thought other people would see me as weak for worrying so much, when perhaps there was really nothing to worry about at all.

When the scan was over, Bernie and I sat in the waiting room. The pictures would be seen by a radiologist and then sent up to Dr Anderson in the Outpatients department. As we sat there, I told Bernie of the sting of the contrast injection and showed her the large bruise on my arm where the needle had gone in. I was feeling sorry for myself. It was simply a bruise. He was a young doctor who did not have the experience and the skill of the blood lady, I told myself. When he had joked with the radiographer, I had felt disregarded, uncared for, that I was the joke; but there had been no intention of that. And, just as I was feeling sorry for myself, I wanted others to feel sorry for me. The bruise became the focus of my anxieties: it was as if I was saying to myself, 'I might be imagining there is something going on in my head, but I am not imagining that bruise; I can see it.' And since others could also see it, I was subconsciously using it as a way of claiming and focusing their attention.

After a while, Bernie and I were directed to the Outpatients building, where Dr Anderson would see us. We sat in the waiting room and watched as a nurse took my pictures into Dr Anderson's room. To have been an invisible presence in there would have been interesting. I would have liked to have heard the discussion between the two doctors. While I was sure that I would be told the 'truth', I knew that the 'truth' as discussed between colleagues would sound different.

Then Bernie and I were called in. It was good to see Dr Anderson again. He immediately showed me the scan pictures, and told me they had revealed only a slight change, and since the bleeding had suggested there was no definite evidence of a tumour, he felt at this

50

stage there was no immediate pressure to interfere. And although a tumour could not be ruled out, Dr Anderson felt it was advisable to wait. I then got out my list of questions, which Dr Anderson immediately took from me. As he carefully went through my questions, he was able to expand on what he had told me. I had asked him to speculate, and to give me informed suggestions as to the cause of my condition. The worst possibility was a brain tumour, and the best, it seemed, was a hamartoma, a kind of congenital tumour such as a malformation of blood vessels. My symptoms, he said, were caused by the swelling bleeding and 'niggling the sensory pathways'.

In my fear, I had decided my hearing on the left side was deteriorating.

'Don't worry. It's probably old age,' he said with customary dry humour.

He reminded me that removal of the swelling was unlikely to be possible: it was too deep. Biopsy, was possible by stereotactic surgery, but, the risks would be high. 'We'll be guided by you – if you can't live with this. I know it's not a lot of fun knowing there is something in your head,' he added kindly. He felt it was safer to wait rather than rush into precipitate action, and said that in a few weeks' time they would do another MRI scan.

Dr Anderson had answered my questions truthfully and directly, and also with great caution and sensitivity; every phase, every nuance was carefully and intelligently weighed. I did not realise this at the time, but it became clear to me later that he did not give anything away that he did not want to. He knew exactly what he was saying, and he assessed with wisdom and intelligence what his patients, certainly this patient, wanted and could cope with.

It was obvious that the situation was not clear-cut: it was a grey area, and a matter of opinion and judgement, not of what was right or wrong. And I trusted Dr Anderson's judgement, and his caution.

As Bernie and I left, I took hold of her arm. She was wearing a dark blue winter coat and I clung tightly to her as we made our way back to the car park. I needed to lean on her, to find some security and comfort. Just as I had become a child in my complaint about the injection and the bruise, and had looked to her then, again I felt small and childlike; I was no longer the articulate questioner who acted as if she had a grip on her situation. The image I hid behind fell away

51

and I became a lost child and looked to Bernie for support. It felt so safe to hold on to her. I was bewildered and my mind was reeling. We had been told so much and yet I felt I knew so little. The scan results were inconclusive: they had shown no obvious sign of change. Deep inside I knew I was disappointed by this. I had known I was feeling worse but there was little objective evidence to prove this. I could not know if I was imagining my own deterioration. I did not know how to make sense of it. If I was not quite able to admit to myself that I was disappointed, then it was certainly not possible for me to talk to anyone else about it: I could hardly say that I had been hoping the scan would show that the swelling was enlarging, and so I had no way of understanding or explaining my disappointment.

By the time we left the hospital car park, I had decided the results were good news. Bernie and I called in at the college where Tony works, and I was able to pass this good news on to him. Tony accepted this as it was given. If I had been able to express my more complex and deeper reaction, he would have accepted that too. He took his cue from me, and supported me in whatever way I was reacting to and dealing with the situation.

This then was the way the outcome of the appointment was passed to friends and family:

'How did your scan go then Viv?'

'Oh fine. There doesn't seem to be much change. So that's good news, really.'

But, unlike the well-worn cliché, no news was not good news; it was a further indefinite suspension into that purgatorial world of limbo and uncertainty. I had convinced myself the results were good, in part because I thought some people would disapprove of me for not being positive, but also because I was beginning to deny the seriousness of my condition; to act, at least on one level, as if it were not life-threatening.

Many of my deeper reactions to it were diverted elsewhere. Psychodynamic theory suggests that at an unconscious level we learn as children that certain emotions are unacceptable in our families – these can vary from family to family – and so we learn to keep these feelings hidden and under control. If a feeling – for example, sorrow or jealousy – is regarded as unacceptable in a family, we internalise this disapproval. We learn not to express it, for to do so would make us unacceptable or unlovable. One of the feelings I had learnt to hide as a child was anger. It was an emotion that was regarded as dangerous and linked with loss of control, a feeling I was too frightened to show. So eventually I learnt not to experience it directly, and although it could occasionally explode out of me, I learnt that it was easier and safer to be the person others wanted me to be. That way I could win their approval and their love.

It might have been reasonable to feel angry about my condition, but I was not able to do so. When friends looked at me and my young children, I could see sadness and pain in their eyes. They would ask, 'Don't you feel angry? This is so unfair.'

And I answered, 'No, I don't.'

Some would say, 'Don't you think, "why me?"'

And I would answer, 'Why not me?'

I experienced this emotion indirectly, in, for example, my reactions to other people's behaviour. In my notebook I cursed the 'idiot who made such a pig's ear of my contrast injection', and I felt greatly irritated by those who would refer to my illness in clichés, who refused to use words like 'tumour' or 'death' or to allow me to use such vocabulary. I said nothing to them but I continued to describe my condition as I wanted, and perhaps almost taunted them with the terms I used. On 15 November, I wrote in my notebook:

I feel anger towards people who say 'Oh no, it can't be a tumour' except they won't use the word itself – they're too scared. I've got to deal with this and I will use this word. I'm not playing games, and I will not pretend. I know they're trying to protect themselves. I also know they believe they're trying to protect me, but I know it's because they won't acknowledge their own fears, their own intimations of mortality. Tough. Fucking tough. This is happening to me, and I will deal with it in my own way. Of course I'm scared – I'm bloody terrified but naming my fears helps to diminish them.

But directing my anger at others was unfair. In a sense, I was blaming them because they did not have to deal with my situation, whereas I had no choice. But there was no reason why anyone else should have to face the implications of my illness. Other people had as much right to suppress or deny any deep feelings as I had to deny and redirect my anger. We were all dealing with deep and powerful emotions.

53

As the end of November approached, I became anxious. I had received no letter of appointment for an MRI scan. I rang the hospital about this and was told there was an eight-week wait for MRI scans and that my scan would be in February. In fact I knew Dr Anderson wanted to leave a gap between scans in order to detect any enlargement of the swelling, but I felt I was getting worse and I was frightened. Driving was becoming slightly difficult. I could only depress the clutch if I consciously and deliberately pushed my left foot down. I still thought I might be imagining my deterioration but I was afraid and felt very vulnerable. I pictured myself at the end of a long NHS queue for an MRI scan and I felt I might be dead by the time I reached the front. Some friends asked us if we wanted to have a scan done privately but I was uneasy about that. I felt medical need, not money, should determine who took precedence in this long queue. I felt I was just another crumbling patient in a crumbling NHS. I felt that those who funded and organised the health service did not give a damn about the patients, although I know that the people who worked within the limitations of the system were committed and compassionate. As I became more worried, I asked Bernie to ring the hospital on my behalf. I felt too upset and vulnerable to do it myself. Bernie rang and talked to the appropriate people and, as a result, I was given an appointment for a scan on 20 January. This felt like a long wait, but I was relieved to have a date. I had hoped it would be before Christmas, but I knew I had to trust Dr Anderson. My fear was that the phone messages were not getting through to him. But, isolated and adrift, I had to wait. As a patient, I had to be patient.

December 1993

During this difficult time, I regularly went to see my GP. Dr Gabriel accepted my need to talk and, while there was no reassurance he could give me, he always gave me his time. I found a kind of reassurance in just being able to refer to a doctor every so often. In his quiet, professional way, he showed great empathy and a deep understanding of the wasteland I had been cast into. I always knew he was there and was accessible.

54

As I counted off the weeks until my next scan, I felt a great need to escape. I could not lose myself in films or television, but I did managed to escape into books. A friend lent me her collection of adventure stories and thrillers, and I buried my head in those. I could hardly bear to come out of them. Facing reality was daunting and exhausting: at times I needed some respite. I did not know what lay ahead, but when I lay awake at three o'clock in the morning, I did not have the courage to contemplate my uncertain future. I would pick up my book, take a sleeping tablet and go into the spare room. Then I fled from reality. Alone, I lost myself in imaginary lives and adventures until my sleeping tablet cloaked my fear.

I no longer played my saxophone. I had neither the energy nor the inclination. Music has been an important part of my life. As a child, I learned to play the piano, and as a teenager, I used to play the guitar and sing. It was the era of the singer-songwriter: Leonard Cohen, Bob Dylan, Joni Mitchell and James Taylor. I loved to sing: music was a means of self-expression for me then. But it was an interest, a creative activity which I had allowed to lapse. As I had grown older, there were other demands on my time and energy. In my late thirties, however, the need to express myself through music was re-awoken, and I decided to learn to play the saxophone. It was an instrument that suited me immediately; while I had no pretensions to ever be a good player, I knew I could be good enough to find enjoyment and fulfilment in playing it. I was drawn to its beauty: to its clear mellow sound and the strength and subtlety of its tone; to its shining golden curves and pearly keys. It is an expressive and personal instrument; it felt like an extension of my voice, a mouthpiece for my deepest feelings. So to pack it away felt as if I was putting away something of myself. I had thought I would have been able to escape into music, to blow away my feelings with every note. But I could not. Perhaps I was frightened to play it in case it aggravated my condition. I do not know. I took it apart and laid it in the case. I unscrewed and collapsed the music stand. I put all my music away. For the moment, perhaps for ever, it was no longer a part of my life.

I kept in regular phone contact with Brenda throughout this time. Whenever we spoke, I felt a lifting of my spirits. For a while, the weight I was carrying would seem less heavy. And the quiet confidence in her voice would renew the sense deep inside me that there was a way through. I also spoke to Philip, the healer I knew in Durham. He, too, was sending out absent healing, and this also helped me. It gave me hope and it kept me going.

Doris, Tony's mother, had stayed with us for most of October and November, and had given us wonderful support. She had collected the children from school and nursery, had given invaluable help with household tasks, and, above all, we had leaned on her solid warmth and kindness. She had left her home and her friends in order to help us, and this assistance was freely given, with love and generosity. As the autumn term drew to a close, Doris returned home for a while and we started to prepare for Christmas.

Tony did almost all of the Christmas shopping. By this time, my left leg was becoming weaker; I had difficulty in walking far, and was no longer able to drive. Tony was carrying an immense load by this time: he was coping with all of the practical jobs and much of the childcare, as well as his own workload. My meagre contribution was to do the Christmas cards. I was left-handed, and although I could hold a pen, I knew my writing was changing: it looked weak and wobbly, but it was still legible. When I commented on it to one friend, she was quick to say, 'Oh, it's fine. There's nothing wrong with it at all.' I was not sure who she was trying to reassure. I knew my writing was different. I knew I had difficulty in using two hands to dress myself. But I accepted her denial. Perhaps I welcomed it.

I included invitations to my fortieth birthday party with the Christmas cards. It was planned for 15 January, a few days after my birthday, and a few days before my MRI scan. The weak and wobbly invitations, written on Dennis the Menace notepaper, went out and were duly replied to. Preparations were under way. I was not going to miss out on the celebration. I had intended for some time to have a party to celebrate my fortieth birthday, and I felt quite determined to go ahead with it. I did not want my condition to alter my plans, and I had no intention of allowing it to do so. In a sense, I was going ahead with the plans for the party out of a need for a diversion, and for something to focus on, and also as a denial of my situation, a refusal to accept that it was serious and life-threatening.

But first there was Christmas. On 11 December we all went to the Christmas Fair at the children's school. It was quite difficult to walk

56

through the crowds of people. I felt distant and uninvolved, except for one sharp moment. I was standing with Josie in the queue to see Father Christmas. She was bouncing up and down with excitement, and I thought, 'This may be the last time I ever do this. I may never take my daughter to see Father Christmas again.' As she sensibly refused to sit on this strange man's knee, I watched my daughter. I looked from afar and imagined her separate life. This was the pain I could not bear. There can be no feeling worse than this: to imagine our children separated and alone, before they are ready.

The following week, my sister came to stay. We saw Stevie at his school Christmas concert, and Josie at her nativity play in the nursery. The junior school had managed to avoid the myths and sentimentality of Christmas, but as I watched the nativity play, and saw Josie, ironically dressed as an angel, I hid at the back and bit my lip, and I fought the feeling. I did not want the pain again. I could not stand the clichés, the cruel construction of Christmas. I had felt angry before we arrived. My anger was like a dam, a huge concrete and steel wall to keep back the fear, the anguish and the tears. I gritted my teeth, clenched my fists and pushed back the raw sorrow. Inside my head, I cursed the social and material construction of joy that is Christmas in the West. I raged at these myths of security and togetherness. I hated them because I was in no position to collude with them. They mocked me with their cosy images of motherhood, of safety and of certainty.

Tony and Louise spent Christmas with us. We had known their parents when we worked in Zambia, and when they came to school in this country, we acted as their guardians. They had frequently spent half-term holidays and weekends with us, and our own children had grown up with them, and saw them almost as big brother and sister. They were now young adults, and we all regarded them as part of our family. They often spent Christmas with us, and it was a delight and a relief that they did so this year.

I found Christmas very difficult. For me, it was a period of limbo while I waited for my next scan, and it was a sharp and constant reminder of what I had to lose. Increasingly over this time, I felt apart from all that was going on around me. I inhabited a different world. Outwardly I was participating in all the activities: I could still feel the joy and the excitement of watching the children open their presents, but I felt disconnected from it. Tony's mother had given us a summer cookery book, and as I looked at the images of summer, I could not imagine how I would be alive by then. I could see no way out. I was clearly getting worse, and the swelling in my brain could not be reached. It seemed an impossible and hopeless situation. I dreaded going to bed at night. I felt locked inside myself and impenetrably alone. I could not escape from my feelings. I lay in bed, enshrouded in darkness and bleak fear. I tried not to take sleeping tablets, but I could not sleep without them. Never have I felt such utter and absolute isolation. I knew nothing at these times. There was no short cut out of such gloom. It could not be fought or struggled against. It was simply there and I had no choice but to live with it.

One morning, I was lying in bed and Louise came up to see me. As she sat on the side of my bed, and we drank coffee together, I wept. Our roles were reversed. When she was a girl, I had sat with her when she was unhappy at school and held her as she cried. Now, at 21, she was holding me. I talked to her about my sorrow and my fear, and then I said, 'And yet, somehow, I have a feeling I will come through this. I don't know how or why. There is no logic or sense to it, but I just have a feeling I'm going to live.'

'You will, Viv. You have been part of my life since I was a child. And you will continue to be part of my life. I know you will.'

She spoke with confidence. They were not words of denial, nor of false reassurance. They came from inside, from her spirit. They were truthful and intelligent. In saying this, Louise gave me something; she touched the spirit deep within me, the part of me that knew I would survive.

I was still taking the Bach Flower Remedies during this time, and I knew that Brenda and Philip were sending me healing. Whether I felt it or not, I knew it was there, just as I knew the love, thoughts and prayers of so many people were there for me.

As December drew to a close, we started making preparations for my party. Friends had offered to do all the food. All I had to do was see to the music. I spent happy hours engrossed in making tapes: soul music, reggae, slow music, rock music, sounds of the sixties and of the seventies. I had always loved to dance and I would not allow my failing leg to prevent me from doing so. I was really looking forward to the party, and I knew I would enjoy it. I felt positive and excited.

January 1994

Philip, the healer, had suggested I contact the Federation of Spiritual Healers to find out if there was someone near to us who could give me contact healing. As a result, Tony and I got in touch with Tom. We went to see him one Sunday afternoon in early January. This quiet, unassuming man gave me healing. I sat in a chair in a warm room; an extension built onto his semi-detached house. A cat wandered through. There was soothing music playing. For half an hour, I sat as Tom held his hands near my head and sent healing. I felt warmth coming from his hands, even though they were not touching me, and I felt calm. Tom knew exactly where the swelling was located and told me, 'This is not cancer. I get a different sensation when I feel cancer is present.' He was making no dogmatic statement nor any claims, but spoke in a modest, matter-of-fact way without arrogance. He had no inner need to reassure me, but was simply telling me what he knew.

Tony and I found this visit, and the subsequent times we saw Tom, both calming and healing. He gave us both what we needed and it was freely given. He had a gift; something he could share, and all we had had to do was to ask for help. Healing of this nature does not wipe away anxiety nor take away fear. Those feelings were present, and could not be denied. I had to live with them. But I knew that the spiritual healing was reaching me and touching my very spirit, my deepest self. I did not float home thinking, 'Oh great, I'm going to be fine;' I still did not know what lay ahead, but somehow I was preparing for it.

We were often asked how our children were coping and usually replied that they seemed fine. We said that we had been truthful with them, that they knew I had a swelling in my brain, and the doctors were not sure what it was. I believed at that time that I had maintained an open and honest dialogue with them. In a situation filled with uncertainty, I had felt it was important that they could be certain of one thing: that I would tell them the truth and not deceive them. But I had not talked to them of my anxieties, or, more importantly, enabled them to express their own fears. As the months had passed since October, I said less and less to them about what was going on. And yet they had tuned into my feelings and were clearly anxious and afraid. At the ages of four and ten, they had an instinctive knowledge of what was happening, a complete and intuitive understanding of what I was facing.

Stevie immersed himself in his many interests, a retreat which was prompted by his more conscious understanding of my condition. His greater independence enabled him to do this. But I think my inability to recognise his deep fear and to meet his needs meant that his feelings were kept inside or projected elsewhere.

Josie's deep feelings were played out in front of my eyes, but while I dimly recognised them, I failed to respond to them. One day in December, Josie was playing with Babby, her panda.

'Mum, Babby's crying, she said.

'Oh, why is that?'

'Babby's crying because Babby's mummy is dead.' A few moments later, she added, 'Babby's name is Josie.'

I was stunned by these words. I did not know what to say. I was too remote, and not sharp enough to grasp what she had been trying to tell me. I failed to see that she had a deep understanding of my illness and the threat that hung over us. I failed to help her address those fears. Her words touched me profoundly but I did not fully comprehend them. Perhaps I did not allow myself to do this. Unconsciously I may have been protecting myself from her pain. My self-deception had known no bounds. My self-absorption had distanced me from my children. I had not recognised their needs. And if I had seen what I was doing, how would I have acted? How should I have acted? I do not know.

On 7 January, Tony and I went to the NEC to see Sting. We had bought the tickets a few months earlier in the hope I would be well enough to go. As we drove into the NEC car park, I wondered if I would be able to walk the considerable distance from the car to the Arena. With my weight carried mainly on one leg, and supported by Tony, we reached the Arena, and found our seats.

'If I ever come here again, I'll probably be in a wheelchair.'

'Well, at least we'll get to the front for Bob Dylan.'

Tony always knew how to make me laugh. I giggled at his dry humour, at his gentle mockery of me and of himself.

'Great,' I replied, lifted out of my self-pity. 'I can hardly wait. Perhaps U2, but Dylan?' I queried in mock amazement.

60

The spotlight figure of Sting appeared on stage and he proceeded to lead his band through rich and varied music. His deep and distant bass guitar carried the audience along. But I was not fully part of the event. I was glad to be there, but I watched with faraway eyes. I listened, but I did not hear the music. I enjoyed it, but it did not touch me. The melodic and the poignant songs almost reached me, but not as I knew they would have done at another time. I was elsewhere. I was one day nearer my MRI scan and whatever it might mean.

A few days later, a friend, Clive, came to visit me. His children attend the same school as ours and he is the local Methodist minister. Clive came with three of the members of his church and conducted a short healing service for me. The simple service was powerful and moving. I had been a little nervous before their arrival: while I had welcomed Clive's offer to come and do the communion, I had worried about feeling awkward and perhaps uncomfortable with the religious language. But none of that mattered. I felt their concern and compassion, and I valued it greatly.

On 12 January, I was 40. Many friends called in to see me that day. We ate pastries and drank coffee. I unwrapped presents and listened to music. My children blew out the candles on my cake, and we continued to make preparations for my party at the weekend.

On the day of the party, many friends came to assist us; they helped to make the house ready and prepared most of the food. On Saturday evening, the children went to stay at a friend's house. People travelled from many places. Durham, Newcastle, Lancashire, London and Northern Ireland. There were old friends – people I had known since I was a teenager – there were friends we had known since our early days in Birmingham in 1972, and others we had met more recently. Alison, my dear and close friend for many years, had flown over from Northern Ireland. She arrived in the early evening. We had not seen each other since August, the time when my symptoms had started, and she seemed shocked when she saw me. She later told me that I had seemed tiny and fragile. I am 5 feet tall and Alison is 5 feet 8 inches, but, she told me, I had never seemed small to her, not until that moment. She helped me to get ready. I could no longer grip anything in my left hand, so Alison helped me to put on my make-up and my little black dress.

The party went well; it was a joyful occasion with dancing and laughter, chatter and conversation, wonderful food and lots to drink. I felt relaxed and found it easy to throw myself into the celebrations. Ironically, had I been well, I would have worried about whether it would be a success, about how so many and such disparate groups of friends would mix. I would have been so tense it would have been difficult for me to enjoy it. But none of this occurred to me. Everyone seemed to have a good time. I was one of the few sober people at the party: I had not drunk anything alcoholic for some months. But that did not matter; I had a wonderful time.

Everyone who came seemed to understand what it meant to me to go ahead with the party. We all entered into the spirit of it and genuinely enjoyed it. In a sense, we were playing parts; we were acting as we would have acted if I had been well, but more so. The mass collusion in my denial was also a show of bravado and defiance; a stubborn refusal to let this thing spoil our fun. But, as such, it was a denial I needed, a communal show of spirit that gave me an important boost.

The next morning, the children returned. It was a relief to see them; the house had started to feel empty and incomplete without them. Immediately, they filled it with their presence. Our friends who had stayed the night left for home and wished me well. We went to see Tom, the healer, that Sunday afternoon. It was four days until my MRI scan.

Alison stayed with me for one week following the party. She would return to Northern Ireland on Sunday 23 January. On Thursday, the twentieth, Bernie called for me at 6.45 a.m. My scan would be at 7.30 a.m. Scanner time is precious, so appointments start early and finish late.

As we drove through the early morning January gloom, the roads were quiet. Bernie parked the car and I looked across to Ward D, its corridor lights showing little activity. I knew the night staff would be completing their shift and the patients would be asleep or drinking tea. We walked across the cold, almost empty car park and entered the silent hospital. As we went into the reception area of the scanner department, a radiographer appeared and welcomed me. There was no one else around except for a cleaner. My appointment was the first of the day.

I handed Bernie my watch and earrings; there was now no metal on my person. I did not know how I felt. I was just ready for the scan. It was the next step and I wanted to get on with it. A few minutes later, I was escorted up the main corridor and out to the car park at the rear of the hospital. I heard again the sonorous rumble of the heavy lorry with its awesome load. Soon, I was lying on the padded table and sliding into the long, narrow tunnel. I closed my eyes, I heard a disembodied voice and then the knock-knock-knocking sound, the buzzing-drilling sounds. I lay there and concentrated on all the people I knew were thinking about me at that moment, as they got out of bed, or ate breakfast. I knew I was not completely alone as I lay inside the scanner. I thought of Brenda, Tom and Philip and the healing they were sending me. I thought of all the friends who lived near to us. Clive had asked many of them to light candles for me that morning. I focused my thoughts on each and every person, and kept my fear at bay. The table slid out. A probe was fitted onto a finger. I never did find out why. I was sent inside for another ten minutes.

When I came out, Bernie took me home. I do not know what I said or how I felt. I think I was operating on a fairly mechanical level. We arrived back at around nine o'clock, just after Tony and the children had left for work and school. I was dazed and confused. Alison fed me with chocolate and coffee. I would know the results of the scan the following Tuesday. I did not wonder what it would show. I knew something was going on inside my head. My left side was progressively weakening. I had some difficulty in swallowing; every so often I would cough and splutter. I frequently bit my tongue, and my sense of taste seemed to be changing slightly. I had stopped reading; the print was jumping around and I could not focus on it. If I was travelling in a car, everything outside seemed to move up and down. This time I did not doubt my own judgement. There was nothing subjective about these symptoms.

Preparing myself for the scan had been very stressful. My main fear had been that it would not take place, and now that it had been done, I felt an enormous sense of relief. This carried me through the rest of the day. In the evening, Tony went out to teach an evening class, and the children were playing upstairs. I was sitting with Alison, and I broke down. I sobbed in her arms. She stroked my hair, as I talked of my fear, of how terrified I was that I was going to die. She sat and listened and she soothed me. My fears had come bursting through. I had not been able to keep them in. Alison held me, she held my fears, and she shared the load.

The following evening, Friday 21 January, Alison and I were due to go to a friend's house, where a group of us would have a Chinese meal. Chris, who had comforted me in September on the day I had received the results of the first brain scan, was to pick us up and drive us over to Sheilagh's house. Chris had been interviewed that day for the headship of a large mixed secondary school in Birmingham. I had been thinking about her and hoping she would be offered the job. I had had a strong feeling that she would. When she arrived to collect us, I opened the door, and looked at her tentatively.

'Yes, I got it!' Shrieks of delight and laughter. The children in that school were fortunate. I knew she would make a difference to the school and to their lives.

We sat in Sheilagh's house. The talk was of education, of local authority advisers and of education officers, of salaries, and of teachers' conditions of service. It was Chris's day and a time for celebration. No one asked me about my MRI scan the day before, and I did not feel able to mention it. I felt they would not want to hear about it, or to know about my fears. I was hurt and upset about this, although it did not surprise me. They would say they were trying to offer me a distraction, to take me out of myself. But I was firmly fixed inside myself: I could not leave and I had nowhere to go.

As we sat and ate our meal, I felt very tired. I was finding it difficult to sit upright on a hard chair – my failing left side would not take its equal share of my weight – so I excused myself from the table and went to sit on a sofa in the lounge. As soon as I was alone, my emotions escaped and quietly I wept. Alison came in to join me. She had sensed my feelings. I cried silently on her shoulder. I did not want the others to know I was upset and could not contain my feelings. Margaret, the friend who had had cancer, came and sat beside us. She, too, knew how I felt. She knew that sometimes sorrow and fear can explode through the social veneer, and that there was no dam great enough to hold back the dark lake of despair. I asked Margaret if she would mind taking Alison and me home. We made our excuses and left. I felt safe once again. As soon as we sat in Margaret's car, I could stop pretending. I should not have gone. I had known I would have to hide what I was feeling. I knew that they felt deeply and cared for me, but that we dealt with emotional experiences in different ways. I understood something of the various mechanisms by which we all protect ourselves. Yet I felt hurt. I felt I was childlike in my inadequacy and could no longer function in an adult world of social skills and concealed emotions.

On Sunday 23 January, Alison left and flew back to Northern Ireland. It was a sad goodbye. We did not know when, or if, we would see each other again.

On Tuesday 25 January, Bernie took me over to the hospital. Dr Anderson had offered to see me when he did his ward round, and to give me the results of the MRI scan then.

Once again, I entered Ward D. I had not visited the ward since my stay in September. The hospital smell, the heat and the atmosphere were the same. The anticipation and the apprehension I felt were sharper. In September I had not known what to expect. This time, I knew what was waiting for me.

Dr Anderson arrived and went into the nurses' office. Then he led us down to one of the bays where he could talk to us privately. I sat on one of the beds and he stood opposite me. A junior doctor stood uncertainly in the doorway. Dr Anderson had watched me as I followed him into the room. He saw my arm hanging limp and my left leg dragging behind. They confirmed what the scan had already shown him. The swelling was slowly increasing in size.

'So, is it a tumour, then?' I asked. 'And can you tell if it's benign or malignant?'

'The angiogram suggested it is unlikely to be highly malignant – it could be a malformation of blood vessels or a low-grade malignant tumour. In the brain you can classify a tumour as benign but in a malignant place. The potential threat is what is happening to the surrounding tissue.'

The problem, it seemed, was the same: the central difficulty was not what the swelling was, but where it was. I asked him what the options were. Complete removal still seemed to be unlikely. A biopsy would be risky, although it would tell them what the swelling was. This then could be followed by radiotherapy. The other option would be to use radiotherapy without a biopsy – blind radiotherapy.

'What would you do?' I asked. 'If you had this swelling in your brain, what would you do?'

'That's a fair question,' he replied and he considered it carefully. He stood and he tried to put himself in my position. Then he answered my question genuinely and honestly. I knew then that he understood what this meant to me, that I had been absolutely right when I had realised on the first appointment that I could trust Dr Anderson.

'I would get an opinion,' he said. 'Is it feasible to remove the lot? How big would the risk be? I might go for blind radiotherapy. But if a surgeon said he could remove it with a twenty per cent chance of little upset, then that might be an acceptable risk.'

'Do you think that's an acceptable risk?' I asked.

'You must work out what figures would be acceptable to you. You will want to know about the nature of the damage, the extent of the risk. It appears to be inoperable, but then I'm not a surgeon.' He said he might refer me for radiotherapy, but first he would consult a surgeon. 'It is time for action,' he added.

I looked at him. 'This is going to kill me, isn't it?' I felt he was unable to answer this unfair question. I think at that moment he felt a sense of hopelessness and helplessness. I wanted to give him a big hug, this warm, good man of humanity and integrity. I knew if he had been talking to a colleague, he would have said that my prospects were not good.

It was hard to leave Dr Anderson that day. He seemed to feel sad. There was nothing more to say and there was no reason for the discussion to continue, but it was difficult to go. How hard it must be for a doctor to give such information to a patient. As Bernie and I walked up the ward, Mary, a nurse I had known in September, asked me if I was all right. I said, 'Yes, fine.' As we left the ward, we passed Dr Tembo and Michael, Dr Anderson's SHO. There was an end-of-term feeling about Michael; he seemed to be bouncing along like a schoolboy beside the sedate figure of Dr Tembo. The junior doctors were due to finish their jobs and would start new posts in February.

We left the hospital, and this time. I felt a sense of relief, almost of exhilaration. It was time for action. Ironically, I was glad. The swelling had enlarged and, ridiculously, I was pleased. T.S. Eliot writes in *East Coker* that 'to be restored our sickness must grow worse', and this was my feeling at this moment. I had emerged from no man's land.

The following day, I contacted BACUP, the cancer information service. I talked to one of their counsellors and asked them to send me information on brain tumours, and on radiotherapy. I needed to do something, to prepare myself for whatever was to come. Surgery seemed to be unlikely so I wanted to find out as much as I could about radiotherapy. I knew I would lose my hair, but I thought of the lovely black velvet hat Doris had bought me for my birthday. I was ready for action and I prepared myself for radiotherapy.

A few days later, a letter arrived to inform me that I would be admitted to the Midland Centre for Neurosurgery and Neurology on 7 February.

I went to see my GP. I needed to talk over the information I had been given and I knew Dr Gabriel would allow me to do this, and would listen as I attempted to make sense of it, and prepare myself for the unknown next step. Physically, I felt quite ill. I was weak, and my vision was changing. I felt pressure in my head, or thought I did. I felt sick, my head ached, and I wondered whether I would last until 7 February. I did not speak of this apprehension, but I later learnt that I was not alone in feeling this way. My deterioration was apparent to others. Tony told me some time later that when we went to bed at night he did not know if he would wake up in the morning and find me dead. But to have expressed such fear then would have been to enter its gaping jaw. It was something neither of us could do.

The weekend before entering hospital was spent in acquiring a cat. Throughout January, we had been looking for an adult cat in need of a home. We all like cats and I felt it would be good if we finally made an effort to get one. In attempting to offer the children a distraction, it is likely I was trying to divert my own attention and to fill the gap in my inadequate handling of their needs. We had been told of a family who wanted a home for their cat, Nuage. He seemed to meet our requirements, although we had reservations about his name. We could not quite envisage opening the back door and calling out 'Nuage'. Tony felt it should be pronounced 'New Age' or alternatively changed to 'Nodger'. However, we were not to become acquainted with Nuage: his owners decided to keep him, though not, I think, because they had caught wind of the change of name.

So, on Saturday 5 February, Tony and Stevie went to visit the RSPCA, where a fine black and white cat chose them as his future owners. They returned with Reg, a confident cat, who soon made his mark. After Tony had cleared this up, we looked at each other and wondered whether we had done the right thing. Reg, however, was unperturbed. He seemed quite settled, so we let him out that evening. Of course, he disappeared, and we spent most of the evening calling 'Reg' out of the back door. This was marginally less embarrassing than shouting for 'Nuage'. Reg refused to come in. Twice he appeared on the garden path, but as soon as Tony went out, he ran off. We gave up the search quite readily. 'You don't care,' Stevie accused us. In a sense, of course, this was true. The whole pantomime felt ridiculous and farcical; our hearts were elsewhere. We gave up and went to bed. The next morning, Tony put some food out on the garden path. Reg appeared and was duly grabbed. Getting a cat the weekend before I went into hospital had proved to be more of a distraction than we had bargained for.

Again, T.S. Eliot seemed to capture the experience: in *Burnt Norton* he writes, 'Distracted from distraction by distraction'. Thus we prepared ourselves for the road ahead. I packed my bag and was ready to move on.

PART THREE

7 February – 1 March 1994

CONNECTIONS

Monday 7 February

The children and I said an understated distant goodbye: it was as if the parting had already been made. Tony took them to school and nursery. When he returned, it was time for us to leave for the hospital. I hugged Doris. She stood by the door and watched us go. There was an unfairness in our leaving her like that. She was alone. The children were at school. She did not have to put herself through this. Yet she was doing so. She was giving us not just practical help but her presence. She did not know what lay ahead, any more than any of us; yet she was willing to lay herself on the line, to expose herself to pain and hurt. I love my mother-in-law. I grew to love her soon after we first met. When I was 21, she made a birthday cake for me. It was the first time anyone had done that. She is strong and constant. I looked back at her and waved. It was easier for me. I was going somewhere; events were unfolding and I would be a full participant, but for the lonely figure behind it was hard. Doris had come to give us support; yet it seemed, that morning, as if we were all deserting her.

Tony and I arrived at the hospital and entered Ward D. I was one of many new arrivals, and was soon shown down to Bay 11, the room next to where I had been in September. The small two-bedded area with its large radiator and high window seemed to stifle me. I stepped out of it into the corridor and gazed longingly across at the car park.

71

By this time, Tony had unpacked my bag and arranged my belongings. My pyjamas lay on my bed but I did not put them on. Above my bed I had seen a pink card. It had my name on it, but not the name of a consultant. I knew from my previous stay that a blue card signified that my consultant was a neurologist. In September, the card had been blue and had on it, my name, and that of Dr Anderson, but this card was pink. The card signified neurosurgery. I was puzzled by this. I was expecting, indeed I thought I was preparing for radiotherapy. But there was no surgeon's name on the card. I wondered what to expect.

A young senior house officer arrived. I had not met him before: the SHOs had just started their new posts. He introduced himself as Pierre. I liked him immediately. He was unthreatening, friendly and kind. He did a neurological examination, checking on my reactions to pinprick, temperature and light, and took a blood sample. It did not occur to me to ask him about the pink card. I was a little dazed and bewildered by it. I did not know was was going on and I did not think of asking.

The patient in the next bed was Daisy. She was very nervous and intimidated both by the atmosphere and by the prospect of whatever she might have to face. We exchanged brief details of our medical conditions. It is amazing how one can disclose such personal information to fellow patients, forgetting that they are, in other respects, complete strangers. Daisy soon began to fuss over me. Tony and I sat out in the corridor, where we could breathe, and talk.

'I miss Judy,' I said to him. 'This is not like last time.' I looked out of the window and could see our car in the car park. I looked down the drive by which we had entered the hospital. If I looked to the right, I could see the entrance to the hospital. The exit from it. I did not know how long I would stay here, nor did I know when, how, or if I would leave. I looked at the exit and I looked at our old blue Golf, a solid, reliable car and a link with home. A way home if I had been able to take it.

Tony went over to college for a couple of hours. Daisy accompanied me to the day room for lunch. Then she accompanied me as I came back. Her needs were great. I lay on my bed and retreated into my Walkman. She went and sat in the corridor with her husband, a kind man, fearful and concerned for his wife. I looked at the photographs on my noticeboard which Tony had pinned up for me.

Then I got out the photographs taken by a friend at my birthday party. He had compiled an album and kindly given it to me. I had brought it in with me, I told everyone, 'to remind me of who I am'. As I looked at myself, with my bright orange hair and my black velvet dress, I saw the image I hid behind. There was no such image now. I was just another dazed figure who did not know what was going to happen. I looked at my friends on that joyful occasion. They had been with me then and I knew they were with me now. Sentimental it may be. But it was so.

Daisy's husband left and she rejoined me. She stayed close. She was clearly very frightened, and this was translated into a need to mother and protect me. I could not escape from her. My Walkman was no defence against her ceaseless chatter. Wherever I went, she seemed to follow. I felt her deep need and her great fear, but I could not help her. I felt as if I wanted to shrug her off. The patient in the next bay was Doreen. She, too, was older than me but she had no need to smother me. She was kind and humorous and easy to be with. She had noticed Daisy's need to adopt me, and was glad to provide a refuge.

Tony returned briefly in the afternoon, and, since I could no longer write, wrote notes to the children for me. I had left presents for them at home, so that when they returned from nursery and school, there would be a distraction. I could not face the thought of them feeling my absence. It was my forlorn and pathetic attempt to mitigate their loss – to make myself feel better. Such circumstances reveal us at our most inept. How could a toy kitten and a digital watch help them to deal with my desertion? They were simply a material expression of my inadequacy, symbols of my sense of helplessness and my inability to take away their pain.

At around four o'clock, Tony went home so that he could spend teatime and early evening with the children. He would return later at about eight o'clock. As I walked down the ward with him, a television was showing children's programmes. I knew Stevie and Josie would be at home watching them. I ached for them; for Stevie's sweet voice and his gentle, sad expression, and for Josie's beautiful face, the feel of her head under my chin and her baby smell.

Chris came in to visit me. She had come straight from work, but this time, unlike in September, she knew what to expect. We sat in the

73

corridor, away from Daisy, and as we talked, I felt as if the place was closing in around me. Daisy's claustrophobic presence and her need of me weighed me down. I told Chris how I felt, and we giggled when I told her that Daisy had offered to help me get ready for bed.

'You've got to get away from her, Viv. This is no good for you.' Chris asserted. I knew she was right, but I did not see how I could escape.

'Let's go and buy some sweets. There's a place by the entrance,' Chris suggested. I held on to her arm and limped along beside her, as we made a temporary escape from Daisy and went in search of chocolate and comfort. As we returned with the goodies, we were joined by Jane and Wendy, two other friends. We arrived back on the ward to find three doctors waiting for me: a registrar and two SHOs. I did not know any of them. The registrar spoke. He did not introduce himself.

'Tomorrow you will have an angiogram. On Wednesday you will have a biopsy.'

'I'm sorry. What? I don't understand,' I feebly muttered.

'Tomorrow you will have an angiogram. Then on Wednesday you will have a biopsy,' he repeated.

Bewildered, I struggled to take in this information. 'A biopsy? I don't understand. I didn't think it was possible. What does Dr Anderson say? What are the risks?'

He talked over me as I stood in confusion.

'What are the risks?' I helplessly repeated.

The three doctors stood over me. The two junior doctors seemed almost as helpless as I felt. The unknown registrar, looked down on me.

'And what job do you do?' he asked. His meaning seemed to be, 'Who do you think you are?' He was clearly an insecure man, that he should find the bewildered questioning of a frightened patient so threatening. Then he produced a consent form for the angiogram, and asked me to sign. It was impossible to sign the form without anything to rest on, so I knelt down and leaned on a chair. It was difficult to kneel down; I had very little strength in my left side. I could not grip the pen, so my signature was little more than a faint wavy line. The three doctors stood and watched me as I did this, and then struggled to my feet again. None of them offered to help. I sensed some feeling of concern from the SHOs, but I think the unknown registrar was enjoying his power.

74

They left and I flopped onto a chair. Chris was appalled by their behaviour, and commented on their body language. I felt shaken and humiliated, a pathetic and passive victim. I would not have expected empathy – doctors have enough to do – but I would have appreciated sensitivity. Wendy cuddled me and comforted me. I felt demeaned and silly, but she said I was right to try and ask a question. I was lost and confused. It seemed that I would be having an angiogram on Tuesday. This was a prospect I did not relish, but I understood it. What was harder to grasp was the talk of a biopsy. I felt I had been given an ultimatum, but no information. There had been no dialogue, and I had no sense of being an equal participant in whatever was to happen next. I did not know what lay ahead and I felt very frightened. I hoped that I would see Dr Anderson or Dr Tembo, his registrar, when they did their ward round on Tuesday afternoon.

After Chris had gone, Wendy and Jane walked down with me to the phone in the foyer at the hospital entrance. I was completely thrown by this turn of events, and wanted to talk to Tony. As we stood and waited for the phone to be free, I leaned on Wendy. She seemed to understand how I felt and how bleak it all seemed. As she cuddled me, I knew she empathised with me, and she gave me great comfort. The difference between sympathy and empathy seems to me to be monumental: in her empathy there was a deep and equal sharing of my feelings. There was a recognition of her own vulnerabilities, a capacity to feel her own pain, and a willingness to enter into my experience and to share some of it. But where there is sympathy, there is also power. With sympathy comes patronage. There is no sharing of experience, but a looking on, perhaps even a looking down on another person. There is separation and distance. When we offer sympathy, we are safe; we take no emotional risk, our own deep feelings can remain unacknowledged as we look on from afar and offer kind words to the object of our pity.

While we were waiting for the phone, Tony arrived. Jane and Wendy left and he took me back to the ward. It was good to see him; to feel his calmness and to lean back on his quiet support. After he had gone, I went into the next bay to visit Doreen. She was chatting to Anne, a patient whose bed was in the Wendy House. Anne told me there were spaces in there and they both suggested I ask the staff if my bed could be moved. This seemed to me to be an ideal solution to my need to escape from Daisy, so when the nurses did the drug round, I explained the situation to them and asked if I could move. They were happy for me to do this, and so while Daisy was watching television, the escape plan was put into action, and I moved into the Wendy House. Anne's easy company and the light and space of the Wendy House were a welcome contrast to the grey, cotton wool feel of Bay 11.

I told Daisy that I had been moved because I had found the other room too warm and stuffy, and she seemed to accept this. I was glad to see that she had found other 'friends', but I felt sad about her. I knew I was selfish and self-absorbed, and that while I had recognised her fears, I had not felt able to meet her needs by allowing her to mother me. I could not play a part for someone else. My instinct was for self-preservation, and that meant preserving a sense of myself. In being self-centred and focusing on myself, my instinct was for survival.

Tuesday 8 February

Tony called in to see me that morning, and we were joined by Clive. He had come to give us his support and the good wishes of everyone in his church. Soon after he arrived, Jean, one of the radiographers, came in. I was to have a CT scan, and it was decided to take me down for it in a wheelchair. I still thought of myself as being able to walk. I think the image I had of myself was slightly at odds with the perceptions of others. I was not able to see what I looked like as I walked. I felt I had a limp – others saw my left arm hanging loosely by my side, and my left leg trailing along behind me. When I saw the wheelchair and came to realise I did need it, I had to face not only a different picture of myself, but also the fact that I was deteriorating rapidly. One month earlier, I had been dancing at my birthday party, albeit with some difficulty. Now I could barely stand. I knew that since the MRI scan in January, my condition had worsened considerably.

As I was wheeled into the scanner department and was greeted by Pauline, I burst into tears. I sobbed, and the two lovely radiographers comforted me. Never have I felt so sorry for myself. I felt helpless and alone. Everything seemed hopeless as I lay there on the scanner table, and I felt there was no way out. I longed for the children, Tony and home, but I felt as if I was already separated from them, from their lives. That I would be forever in the scanner, forever in the hospital, forever far away. Forever, never to be part of their lives.

After the first part of the scan, a doctor came in to do the contrast injection. She was a very pleasant and efficient young woman. As she skilfully and painlessly injected the contrast medium into my right arm, we chatted easily. I had suppressed my feelings of despair. They had escaped for a few minutes and now I was firmly sitting on them. I had barely been able to tolerate such raw anguish. I had not been able to contain these feelings, but nor could I bear to experience them. It was easier to focus my attention on a friendly chat with a doctor than to feel such pain and desolation.

After the scan, I was told they would take me straight up to the X-ray department for the angiogram. I was briefly alarmed by this but mainly relieved as it gave me less time to worry about it. I was loaded back into the wheelchair and swiftly taken up to X-ray. Before I had time to think about it, the radiographers were preparing me for the angiogram. Then the radiologist came and introduced himself. Dr Webb told me that although we had not met, he knew my case well. I felt a scratch on the back of my hand; I do not know what it was but I felt quite light-hearted after it. Then he injected local anaesthetic into the right side of my groin, both above and below the femoral artery, and inserted a catheter into the artery. I felt very little pain as he did this. He had an air of brisk professionalism about him, and a very direct and efficient manner. I liked him. After the pictures had been taken of the cerebral arteries, I asked him if he would talk about biopsy versus blind radiotherapy. It seemed to me that no definite decision had been made at that stage as to what to do. Up-to-date information was still being gathered and discussion was continuing between the doctors.

As Dr Webb stood with his elbow in my groin, applying pressure to the punctured artery, he gave me an analytical and dispassionate view of the two options. He seemed to feel that a biopsy was possible, and that while it carried some risk, was preferable to blind radiotherapy, which would change the nature of the swelling, and in doing so, mask the evidence. I found Dr Webb's cool, clinical appraisal of my case very helpful. Up till then, my head had been reeling. I had felt completely in the dark and there had been no opportunity to talk to anyone, apart from Dr Kamen, the registrar from the night before. This was the first time I had been able to ask about the possibility of surgery, and Dr Webb's objective and academic way of giving his views was exactly what I needed. I did not want ultimatums, but nor was I looking for soothing words as a palliative to my feelings or vague generalisations which avoided the issue. I understood that the doctors were not yet ready to commit themselves to a course of action, but I greatly appreciated the way Dr Webb talked to me that day. I felt he treated me as a person, and as an equal. For a while, he stood, and we talked about working in Africa. He, too, had spent some time in central Africa, and we discussed the scandal of the powdered milk companies and the promotion of their products in the developing world.

When the artery had stopped bleeding, I was carefully lifted from the X-ray table onto my bed, which had been brought up from the ward. I was wheeled back to the ward, where Tony was waiting for me. I was eager to tell him about the conversation with Dr Webb. I felt excited and animated as I did this, and that I had moved away from the despair I had experienced as I went in for the CT scan. In giving me something to think about, and a sense of being included in a discussion of my case, Dr Webb had lifted my spirits. I knew I was suppressing and denying my fears, but at the same time I had a sense of being involved, and of being active. I no longer felt like the passive victim of the night before, and this was a way of coping, a way of protecting myself from such dark feelings.

I had to lie flat for the rest of that day, but, unlike in September, when the sedatives I had been given had made me feel cut off and adrift, this time I was still part of what was going on around me. I was able to chat to Tony and to Anne in the bed opposite.

Dr Tembo, Dr Anderson's registrar, did his ward round that afternoon. I was disappointed not to see Dr Anderson but it was good to see Dr Tembo. I had not seen him to talk to since he had carried out the unenviable task of breaking the bad news to me in September. There was clearly nothing he could tell me at this stage, but I asked after Dr Anderson and said I would like to talk to him, if it were possible. Now that I had taken in the fact I had been referred to a neurosurgeon, and that there was a possibility of a biopsy, I felt a strong need to hear Dr Anderson's opinion. I felt safe and secure with him, and while I knew that any course of action was a question of judgement and not of right or wrong, I felt that I wanted the green light from him.

During the evening, Brenda called in to see me. As always, she lifted my spirits. She told me, 'You will be well again,' and in the way she said it, and at a spiritual level, I knew it was true. I still had great fear and doubt, but at a level beyond that, underlying it, was a feeling that I would come through. Without the spiritual healing, all my hope would have long gone.

Wednesday 9 February

On Wednesday I had a feeling of waiting; I was anxious and a little impatient. However, there seemed to be a pace and a sense to the way in which events were slowly, but inexorably, unfolding. I did not see it then, but there was meaning and order to everything that was happening. Every event, every feeling, was a preparation for each subsequent stage. From the confusion and despair of Monday night and Tuesday morning to the logic and the rationale of Dr Webb, from the hope that seeing Brenda had rekindled in me to whatever was to happen next. I had a sense of moving on. I had been told that later that day I would meet Mr Meyer, the consultant neurosurgeon to whom I had been referred. I was curious to meet him and anxious. I had grown to trust Dr Anderson and was not sure whether I would experience the same degree of trust in a different doctor.

Later that afternoon, I was told that Mr Meyer had arrived on the ward and would be coming down to see me. I lay on my bed in the Wendy House, took out the earphones of my Walkman and anticipated his arrival. A few minutes later he came in, a smartly dressed man in a white shirt, dark suit and tie, and steel-rimmed glasses. He greeted me with a firm, strong handshake and with a slight Australian accent introduced himself as Carl Meyer. Then he explained to me, clearly and logically, the options that were available for my treatment. He told me that radiotherapy would slow down the advance of the swelling, but would also do some damage to surrounding brain tissue, and that the extent of this damage could not be precisely predicted.

79

The radiotherapy would not destroy the lesion. It would work slowly and would, at best, contain the swelling, which was still bleeding.

There was however, the possibility of surgery; this would be done stereotactically, and would involve having a steel frame screwed into my head. Along the frame are calibrations which enable precise co-ordinates to be taken of the position of the lesion in the brain. These, together with the three-dimensional constructions of the brain obtained through CT scanning and angiography, would enable a path to be taken through the brain which carried as low a risk as possible to healthy brain tissue. The fitting of the frame, I was told, would involve a feeling of tremendous pressure, but not of pain, and then, under local anaesthetic, a biopsy would be taken by inserting a needle through the skull and extracting a small amount of the lesion. The risk involved in doing this was high; there was the possibility of damage to surrounding tissue, and also a risk of haemorrhage from the procedure itself. In addition, it was not always possible with biopsy done this way, to ensure that the right bit of tissue was obtained.

A third option was a biopsy done at close range. This was a slim possibility as it carried a very high risk. It would involve a craniotomy; under general anaesthetic, a plate of bone would be removed from my skull, and an attempt would be made to take a biopsy from the swelling. There was also, it seemed, a slight chance that complete removal might be possible, although this seemed unlikely. The operation, he told me, would be the following week. 'You need time to get to know me, as you've got to know Dr Anderson.' And with a handshake this courteous and charming man left.

There was a lot of information for me to take in. Just a few days earlier, I had been expecting radiotherapy, and now, it seemed, surgery in one form or another was an option; an option which obviously interested me, but was also alarming. I needed to talk to Dr Anderson. I wanted to hear his opinion. I was glad that Mr Meyer had recognised the trust I had in Dr Anderson, and that such trust was a necessary part of the relationship between patient and doctor. I feel it does not come simply from a knowledge that a patient might have of a doctor's expertise or experience, but is a deeper trust which arises from the relationship itself, from each person's sense of the other.

The relationships I had with staff were becoming increasingly important to me. I had felt a strong, almost maternal sense of security from Jean and Pauline, the two radiographers with whom I had most contact. The staff on Ward D were, I felt, quite exceptional, and it was easy to build up strong and friendly relationships with them. Everyone on the ward – cleaners, nurses, auxiliaries, sisters – seemed to relate to each patient as an individual. Each staff member had her/his own particular strengths. They were all approachable and easy to talk to, relaxed and friendly. Each member of staff wore a name badge, and it felt important to me to be able to use their names. It was a way of establishing a personal relationship, of going beyond the uniform. It gave me a sense of each one as a person, a means of making genuine contact, and from this I gained a sense of myself; I felt recognised and validated. I felt valued, that I mattered, and that each of the staff I got to know mattered too. This helped to give meaning to being in hospital. Without these relationships and a sense of involvement, the days would have felt empty and devoid of anything worthwhile. On Ward D, I felt cared for, and I felt this from everyone, from the domestic staff who changed the jug of water on my locker and cleaned the ward to the consultants who were responsible for my care.

It seemed to me to be wrong that a hospital such as Midland Centre for Neurosurgery and Neurology should be closing. It was evident that there was great sadness and concern about its impending closure: there was fear about jobs and about the loss of a hospital with a tradition and a reputation for excellence. It seemed that decisions had been made about its future without any awareness of the real quality of the place. That it was a centre of great expertise was evident, and perhaps some of its qualities could be moved elsewhere, but the heart and soul of the hospital could not be removed and transplanted into another location. It had grown and evolved over a period of time. The quality of care which was so special in MCNN derived not just from the right number of efficient and well-trained staff, but from the depth of commitment and humanity, the combined sense of purpose and the morale of each and every member of staff. The ethos of a hospital is not something that can be measured in economic terms, and in fact is not quantifiable at all.

That evening, many friends came in to see me; several of them had not yet seen the photographs of my birthday party. As they looked at the pictures of themselves laughing and dancing, Ange produced a photograph of me taken about four years earlier. 'You said you wanted to be reminded of who you are!' she said. The photograph had been taken one drunken evening when Ange, Treas and I had returned to Ange's house, and after a few headstands in her hall, had decided to go out roller skating. Ange and Treas had decided I should wear Ange's 12-year-old daughter's bridesmaid dress for this escapade. It was a pale blue satin garment, trimmed with lace and pearly buttons. So, at two o'clock in the morning, we had gone out, and Ange and I had roller skated up and down her road. I looked at the photograph of myself in the bizarre outfit, and remembered the occasion; how we had giggled, how we had disturbed her neighbours. It seemed a long time ago. But it was a 'me' I recognised: a Peter Pan figure, a playful mischievous person. I knew that part of me still existed, and it was good to be reminded of it.

'The corridor of this ward would be brilliant for roller skating down. It's so smooth. You could go really fast. Do a few twirls on the way,' I fantasised. 'The patients could be a bit of a problem though – they might get in the way,' I joked, trying to pretend I was not one of them, hiding once again behind a false image of myself. In mocking those who were patients, and distancing myself from them, I was avoiding the truth. In my dreams and my silly jokes, I was very consciously deceiving myself, pretending none of this was happening. My light-hearted self-deception fooled no one. I was frightened, and it was apparent to everyone.

Thursday 10 February

I lay in bed that morning, listened to music, chatted to Anne in the bed opposite and wondered what was going to happen next. The conversation with Mr Meyer the day before had given me a glimpse of possibilities. There was nothing definite, but the path ahead seemed to be opening up. Tony called in to see me, and not long after, I heard the deep sound of a voice I recognised. Dr Anderson's tones seemed to permeate and underlie all of the other sounds of the ward. When he appeared, he was dressed in casual outdoor clothes. It was wonderful to see him. It seemed as if he had come in especially to see me, and he told me he was going away the next day for a week of skiing.

82

'Thank you for coming in. It's lovely to see you. So what do you think? What's all this about a biopsy?' I asked.

'Well, I've talked to Mr Meyer and he has persuaded me it is technically possible to do it. I pushed him hard. I told him, "You could paralyse that wee girl," but he has convinced me that there is a way of doing a biopsy at close range. It will mean a craniotomy. If, when they get in there, they find there is a chance of removal, then that might give you some prospect of improvement.'

'I'm amazed,' I said. 'I thought there were no options left.'

'Yes, it was looking that way. This is a bonus. Surgery looked unlikely, but Mr Meyer has persuaded me that it is possible. A craniotomy would mean you won't be able to drive.'

'That's the least of my worries,' I commented.

He nodded. 'If removal is not possible,' he continued, 'we would at least be able to get a piece of tissue, to find out what it is.' Then he added, 'And you can ask me how long you've got.'

'Thank you,' I said. This, I knew, was the answer to my question on 25 January, 'Is this going to kill me?' I was glad Dr Anderson had answered me. I respected him for it. I was not shocked to hear this. I was just glad that he had answered me truthfully. I would not have expected anything less from him. In January I had pushed him to give me his opinion – I simply had to know what I was facing. Whether I could have asked such questions without the knowledge Brenda had given me, is, of course, a different matter. I do not know. Tony then asked Dr Anderson what he could say to friends and family when they phoned: he needed a succinct way of passing on the information we had been given.

'Say that it's a lump in the brain which has bled and grown, that we don't know exactly what it is.' He said that it seemed to be a cluster of abnormal blood vessels, the edge of which had thickened. A biopsy would show whether the cells of this were cancerous or not.

I felt that this was hopeful news: surgery would give me a chance, the impasse had now been cleared. I had the impression that Dr Anderson had played devil's advocate with Mr Meyer, and had made him argue the case for surgery, and I felt that if Dr Anderson, with his caution and patience, had been convinced that it was a chance worth taking, then I was also convinced. It seemed I had been given the green light I wanted. The fact that the swelling was still bleeding and enlarging had shown that it was 'time for action' – Dr Anderson's words in January – action that would have to be taken soon. The operation would be the following week, when Dr Anderson was away.

As he left, I said, 'Have a good holiday. Don't fall down any mountains.'

He patted his round tummy and replied, 'I've got plenty of padding if I do.'

I wondered if I would ever see him again.

Later in the day, Pierre, Mr Meyer's houseman, came in to see me. There was almost an air of excitement about him as he told me the operation was definitely on for the following week, probably the Wednesday. We were told that Mr Meyer would come in to see us on Friday afternoon to talk about it.

The pace seemed to be increasing. With every day, every extra piece of information, every shift in emphasis, there was something more to assimilate and to adjust to. Sometimes I felt as if I was being buffeted this way and that by gale-force winds, and I had no sooner regained my balance than I was hit by another gust. But with each one I was moving forward. It was a struggle to keep standing in the face of these powerful forces. I did not know where they were taking me, but I knew that I was going. There was no turning back, no standing still and no sheltering from the storm. I felt tiny, and frightened and vulnerable. I was dazed. I felt as if I was being whipped up into the air by a tornado, then dropped back down again. I was spinning round and round, dizzy and confused, carried along by forces over which I had no control, forces that were beyond me. I had to accept this, let it happen, but keep moving. The one thing I could not do was to curl up in a ball and hide away. I had to go with the pace of events, be carried along by their momentum. Keep going. Always keep going.

Yet in the midst of this turbulence there existed a 'still, small voice of calm'; the eye of the storm. I could not explain it. It was in me, deep within me, and it was beyond me. It was a certainty, a confidence that as events escalated, I was heading in the right direction, and that I would come through. It was a deeply spiritual feeling – unlike anything I had experienced in my life. I told several people that I had a feeling that I would survive. I knew that in medical terms, the odds were heavily stacked against me, and I still had my fears. I seemed to be operating at different levels: there was the inner core of certainty, the spiritual level at which I knew I was going to live, but there was also the rational level. Medically and logically, my chances were slim and so, associated with that knowledge, there was fear, great fear, and at times despair. The psychological mechanisms of coping were brought into play to deal with these often intolerable feelings, and at this time, just as over the preceding months, I protected myself through such strategies as projection, repression and denial.

That evening, during visiting time, a friend brought in some brochures from a health farm. A few weeks earlier, a group of us, all women friends, had talked about how we would love a day out, or a weekend, at one of these places. It had appealed to me particularly, and Debbie had sent off for information. She had done this out of kindness to me. She had seen that this was a faraway dream, that I had been imagining myself to be someone else, someone fit and healthy. I did not realise I had been doing this. My denial and self-deception were so great, I had really imagined I would be able to go away with my friends for the weekend. As we all perused the glossy brochure, and groaned at the price list, I genuinely believed I would be able to go. It seemed a good idea. It seemed realistic. Then I said, seriously and in a matter-of-fact way, 'Maybe don't arrange it yet. Let's wait until I'm better,' and saw a cloud pass over Debbie's face. I must have registered this cloud at a semi-conscious level, but I did not take in its implications at that time. I genuinely thought I would be going away with my friends on this trip. I had no idea that I was deceiving myself. I was acting as if I was fit and well, or soon would be. I think perhaps I needed some self-deception at this stage. It was a way of coping, of looking ahead, albeit unrealistically, of temporary escape from uncertain and terrifying reality. The cloud which had passed over Debbie's face was a cloud of sadness, of concern for me, a cloud of realisation that I might not get well at all, a cloud that showed she knew that I might die. I am glad she inadvertently revealed that feeling to me; even though I was not fully able to pick it up at the time.

Friday 11 February

I sat on the side of my bed on Friday morning. Anne, who had been in the bed opposite, was going home that day, and I knew there was a slight possibility that I would be able to go home for the weekend. The other patient in the Wendy House was Julie, a woman in her early twenties who had multiple sclerosis. I felt that she had suffered a lot in her life, that the odds had been stacked against her, and that for her, life had been a struggle for survival. Her appearance was cheerful and bright, but there was a brittle edge to it; a thin, shiny, transparent shell that served its purpose, that afforded her some protection in the outside world. But there are times when none of us can fully protect ourselves, when circumstances will strip us bare and shatter our shells and our illusions, when we are revealed, and when we will reveal ourselves.

Suddenly, and seemingly out of the blue, Julie appeared and sat down beside me. She put her head on my shoulder and she sobbed. She sobbed and she shook. She clung to me and cried her heart out. I put my arms round her as this tide of emotion flooded from her. As she opened her heart to me and entrusted me with her fears and her worries for her future, I felt humbled and privileged. She sobbed for herself, and also for me. Then she said, 'You're gonna be all right, Viv. I know you are. You are strong. You will come through this.' The words, which came straight from her heart and from her spirit, were honest and clear and with them she gave me strength.

Later that morning, I was chatting with Denise, one of the auxiliary nurses; she is a warm and compassionate woman who showed great empathy for the patients. I had said to her earlier in the week that I had a feeling I was going to survive, and she told me that she felt I would, that I had strength. I do not think I was strong at all – I did not feel strong – but in what they said to me and the way they said it, both Denise and Julie fuelled my inner feeling and boosted my confidence. Any strength that was in me came from a spiritual source and was fed by the intuition, love and spirituality of people around me.

In the early afternoon, I was visited by Maggie from the Neurophysiology department. She had come to do an ECG in preparation for the operation the following week. As she stuck on heart monitor pads and connected them up to her machine, we chatted. She lived, it seemed, in the same area of Birmingham as me. We talked about secondary schools in that area – my son was 18 months away from finishing primary education, and her children went to one of our neighbouring schools. It was good to talk about my other concerns, everyday but nevertheless important matters, and to remember that in the midst of issues of life and death there are other things to think about. I enjoyed this conversation; it distracted me, but it also brought me back to earth. The question of secondary transfer for our son and indeed the issues of an inadequate education system were important and firmly rooted in the here and now. It was useful to be reminded of this.

After Maggie had gone, Tony arrived and we packed some of my belongings in anticipation of my being let out for the weekend. Then we sat in the armchairs in the corridor, just outside the Wendy House, to await the arrival of Mr Meyer. It was an anxious time; I was anxious and eager to go home, I was anxious about what he would say, I was just anxious. Tony read a book. I listened to a tape on my Walkman. Every so often I would take out the earpieces, listen to the sounds in the corridor, exchange a few brief words with a nurse or another patient, stand up, walk a few steps, sit down, go to the bathroom, listen to some music again, look down the corridor towards the doors, flick through a magazine, swallow, exchange a few words with Tony, listen to a tape, have a cup of tea. And so on.

At about 4.30, Mr Meyer came through the doors. He called in briefly at the office and then, accompanied by Valerie, the sister on duty, he came down to see us. He introduced himself to Tony and shook hands with both of us. Then he pulled up a chair and sat opposite us. Clearly and logically, Mr Meyer explained to us what was happening, what the operation would involve and what the risks were. He reminded us that the swelling had bled twice, was growing and that it could bleed again. Blind radiotherapy, he said, might stop things advancing, but 'it is unlikely to make you better'. Using the analogy of a mushroom, he drew a sketch and told me that the lesion was at the very top of its stalk, the brainstem. 'It's right there in the clockwork, in the core of the brain, and only just within the limits of operability; it's almost inaccessible.'

We listened and tried to take in this information. It was not new – I had heard it in September – but the reality of it was so massive that I was still shocked every time I heard it.

'The reason for the operation is to find out about something which has the potency to kill you. The merits of surgery are that we can find out through biopsy if it's a slowly growing tumour, and there is the

87

possibility of removal. But the risks are high. If I could guarantee you another five years, then such risks might not be worth taking. But you are young. You have children.' He did not say it, but I suspected that without such direct intervention I would be lucky to have weeks let alone years.

At some point Julie drifted down the corridor. She looked quite lost and stopped by us. I think she asked me to fasten a button on the top of her jumper. In a daze, I was ready to comply. Valerie, the sister, sensitively and firmly intervened. 'Julie, could you wait? Viv's talking to her consultant.' She gently guided her away. Valerie returned and I nodded my thanks.

Mr Meyer continued. He told us the operation would be done with stereotactic guidance and would involve the removal of a plate of bone from either the right side or the top right of my head, although the final decision on the approach would be made in the light of information yet to be gathered: there could be a brain scan the day before the operation.

'So what are the risks?' I asked.

Mr Meyer, unlike the registrar Dr Kamen earlier in the week, was undaunted by such a question. As a surgeon, it was his job and his responsibility to point out every risk. And this he did. With clarity and precision, he told me that the risks were as follows: an epileptic tendency, intensification of my existing symptoms, and the possibility of chronic and intractable pain, hemiplegia of the left side, visual problems such as a squint and double vision, and almost certainly the loss of my left visual field. There was a risk of infection, as with any surgery, and the risk of further haemorrhage both during and after the operation.

'And death?' I asked. It was a rhetorical question. I asked it twice, but I expected no answer. There was a slight inclination of his head. I looked at the floor. Slowly, I shook my head. 'This is grim,' I muttered to myself.

I knew that I could die during the operation but I also knew that I would certainly die if it was not done. There was no choice to make. I had nothing to lose, but there was a slight possibility I had something to gain. If Mr Meyer was prepared to take the risk, then so was I. 'We go ahead, then,' I mumbled. 'When will it be?'

'Thursday, next week. It was going to be Wednesday, but I want to be available for the period immediately after the operation, and I can't do that on Wednesday. Now, do you have any questions?'

Tony produced a list of questions, most of which Mr Meyer had already answered. 'How long will the operation take?' Tony asked.

'About six hours.'

'How will I feel after it, both immediately and then later?' I asked.

'There's likely to be some intensification of the symptoms, so initially you'll feel worse, but then you may feel a little better. Is there anything else you want to ask?'

'I think that's everything. I can't think of anything else at the moment.' Then I asked, 'Can I go home for the weekend? I want to spend some time with my children.'

'Yes, of course you can. You can come back in on Tuesday morning, about ten o'clock.'

'Thank you. I just want some time with my children,' I repeated, more to myself than to Mr Meyer.

'Yes. Now if there's anything else you want to ask me, anything at all, then just ring the ward sister and she'll let me know.' He turned to Valerie. 'I'll be in Outpatients on Monday afternoon.'

He stood up and we shook hands. Then he said, 'I will move heaven and earth to give you the best chance of coming through this.' He left, followed by Valerie.

I just sat. I hardly knew where I was. When Valerie returned, she suggested that we go and sit in the nurses' rest room. She led us down to a cosy little room next door to the office. I sat on the small pink sofa. Valerie put the kettle on for us and left us alone for as long as we needed. Tony made some tea. I sat. Then I started to cry. I had been told nothing I did not already know. Everything I had been told, I needed to know, I needed to face. But it was still very hard. There seemed to be few grounds for hope. If ever I had had to face the fact that I might die, it was then. And that moment of truth was desperate and bleak. It was a truth that I could not turn away from. I could neither avoid it nor deny it. We sat in the little room with its rosy-pink furnishings and pictures of flowers on the wall, and sipped our hot tea. Tony sat in silence, the heavy weight of it all pushing down on him. I sat and cried. I thought of the children. I wanted to be at home with them. But I had no strength to move. We sat there, and after a while, Tony went down to collect my bag. Then he came back for me. I pushed myself up onto my feet, and we went into the office to let Valerie know we were leaving. As I hugged her, I started to cry again.

She could barely speak and there were tears in her eyes. I knew how strongly she felt for us. I could feel her deep compassion.

I held on to Tony's arm as we slowly made our way out of the ward. As we left, Mr Meyer passed us. He walked for a few brief steps alongside us, and there was a moment of awkwardness.

'Have you finished for the day?' I asked. I did not know what else to say, so I took refuge in a meaningless question.

He said, 'No,' and darted off to the left, taking a short cut through the lecture theatre.

We dragged ourselves down to the entrance. Tony sat me on a chair in the foyer while he went to bring the car right up to the door. Then he helped me into it.

We drove home through the rush hour, everything around us so ordinary and yet unreal. We passed a bathroom showroom on the Dudley Road, its mundane and functional displays for some reason grabbing my attention. Even in the midst of such drama, we are reminded that the world goes on: people buy new bathroom suites. For most of our lives, it is the undramatic which claims our attention. Perhaps it is safer that way.

As we sit in the heavy traffic, I say to Tony, 'If I die, I want you to feel able and free to meet someone else. As long as she is someone who cares about the children.'

He makes no reply. He concentrates on driving, on negotiating our way through the heavy traffic. I tell him which of my close friends I want to be involved with the children. I need to say these things. Tony needs to get us safely home. 'I don't think I'm going to die. But I have to say these things,' I say.

We drive down from Five Ways roundabout, stop at the lights and then head up past the Central Mosque. We queue to join the Stratford Road, then the Warwick Road. As we approach home, I stop talking. I prepare myself for our arrival, for seeing the children. I try to anticipate how I will feel but I do not know. I cannot imagine. I do not know where I am, and I do not know what is happening. It is just too big.

We arrived home. Doris opened the door and let us in. The house was unexpectedly quiet. My sister Val had taken the children out to McDonald's. Doris made us some tea and, as we sat, I told her what we had been told.

90

'Mum, if I die, will you look after Tony and the children?' What an intolerable burden to have placed on my dear mother-in-law. How could I have asked it of her? I can only think I needed to say it. To name my fear and to voice it. Just as I had done in the car with Tony. These were not well thought out, considered words. They were an expression of my need to say what I feared most. To name what I could barely tolerate. The only way I could confront my fear was with words. They were the only weapon I had. When Mr Meyer had detailed the risks of the operation, I had asked, 'And death?' I could not stop myself. It was as if I was driven to ask the question. I needed to hear myself say the word that I feared most. I was testing myself, and in a sense I was testing others.

In testing myself, I was making myself face the possibility of my death. Somehow I had to feel the fear at its worst in order to move through it; and then I could look back at it and say, 'I know you. I know your name.' My words were the only means of control I had. Without them, I would have felt more lost, more helpless.

In testing others, I was also perhaps establishing some small degree of control – I might have no power over my destiny, but at least I could show that I was aware of what I was facing. By asking Dr Anderson, 'Is this going to kill me?' and Mr Meyer, 'And death?', maybe I was just trying to get in first, to find some means of control. Both Dr Anderson and Mr Meyer were quite exceptional in the way they engaged in honest and equal dialogue with me, and accepted my need to ask questions which were often uncomfortable and difficult to answer. I think, as a patient, I probably demanded a lot of them and gave them both quite a hard time.

Val returned with the children, who were excited and delighted to see me, but at the same time wary and uncertain. I was no longer part of their everyday lives. Their normality had been turned upside down, they were adjusting to being looked after by other adults, and in some ways, my presence was disruptive; it reminded them that I was not part of their normal lives, and it threatened any sort of equilibrium they had found.

I think such feelings must have been deeply bewildering for them. It is difficult for many of us to manage ambivalence. And often, instead of understanding or accepting the co-existence of contradictory feelings, we split them; we may idealise someone or depict them as all bad, or we may simplify our responses to a situation in order to make it seem more manageable. But life is not a Disney film; it is infinitely more complex. And I think there was a lot going on between the children and me that was both complex and contradictory. There was an emotional distance between us; we inhabited different worlds. It was safer to do this than to connect with each other, because just below the surface was a dark lake of fear, a deep pain, that we could hardly bear to acknowledge. The children knew that I was going to have an operation in which they would try to remove the 'thing' in my head, but we did not tell them how risky it was. In fact I cannot remember telling them anything at all. I think I was so wrapped up in my own concerns that I did not consciously think about what I should do, or how I should deal with their emotional needs. And yet, I think they both knew that we were coming to the crunch. They instinctively understood exactly what was going on. That evening, Stevie came into the room where I was sitting; he could barely look at me and was unable to meet my eyes. The pain on his face and behind his eyes was immense. I wanted to take that pain away from my son, and there was nothing I could do. Absolutely nothing. He left the room, and went to talk to Tony. He had reached a point where it was as if he was impelled to demand that the words be spoken. With great courage, my ten-year-old son said to his dad, 'Mum might die, mightn't she?' It was as if he was driven to ask this, to push Tony as hard as he could. Stevie needed to hear the words he feared so much.

Tony answered him truthfully, 'Yes, she might. She may come through it – this operation could save her life. But yes, she might die.'

I do not think it would have been possible for Stevie to have asked this question of me. It would have been too painful for us both; we were almost avoiding each other.

I rang my father in Durham that evening, and told him that they would be operating the following week. I asked him if he would come down to Birmingham the next day. I felt a deep childlike need for my dad. Like a little girl, I cried on the phone to him. I just could not keep it in. I did not spell out the risk of the operation to him: there was no need to. But I felt that if I did not see him that weekend, I might never see him again. And I think he felt the same. This was all unspoken, but I knew it was important to see him, and I knew nothing and no one would have stopped him coming.

I asked Tony to ring Bernie to ask her if she would call to see me. I felt I needed to talk to her, to go over with her what we had been told, and just to lean on her. Her support was something we had both come to value greatly.

Shortly before Bernie was due to arrive, Ange and Treas unexpectedly called at the house. In September, when they had visited me in hospital, I had felt that I had to keep my emotions hidden. This option was not open to me that Friday night. I could keep nothing hidden. My distress was pouring out of me. Treas and Ange came in and sat with me, and as I told them how hopeless it all seemed, and sobbed my way through the account, they were wonderful. They sat with me and they also cried, and in doing so, showed me how much they cared.

When Bernie arrived, she gave me reassurance and support. She reminded me that surgeons have to be cautious and have to err on the negative side, and without giving me false hope, she enabled me to feel that there still was some hope. In addition to this, she passed onto me something of her stillness and deep calm; this was more than just comforting, it was also healing.

During the evening, Brenda rang, and as I spoke to her and expressed my despair, I felt once again the inner knowledge that was the source of my hope, and I knew there was a way through. The voice inside telling me that I would survive was faint, but could just about be heard; my balance on the tightrope between hope and despair was precarious, but it also seemed that it was at my bleakest moments that I could touch that spirit within and beyond me. It was as if I had to experience that darkness, and to face the possibility of dying, in order to know that I would live. When Mr Meyer had described the risks of surgery, I had initially felt that he had left me with little hope, but in fact this was not the case. What he had done was to fully prepare me for what I had to face, and then in saying, 'I will move heaven and earth to give you the best chance of coming through this,' he had given me hope and had shown me that if there was a way through, he would take it.

Saturday 12 – Sunday 13 February

When my dad arrived from Durham, it seemed absolutely right that he had come. I had felt no apprehension and no misgivings about

93

asking him to do so. The minute he walked through the door and hugged me, I could feel his great strength and how much it meant to him to be present. Although it has always been difficult for me to talk openly with him about emotional matters and about the implications of serious illness – these are areas that we deal with in different ways – I think, at those moments when the truth has been very clear, my dad has an honesty of emotional expression which can break through the language of denial. There was no awkwardness, no skirting round the truth, almost no need to talk at all. My dad fully understood what I was facing and how frightened I was, and with his great love gave me what I needed. His feeling that I would come through the operation came straight from his heart. There were no false words of hope and no pretence, just his sense that I would indeed survive. He could have given me nothing more.

On Sunday afternoon the sky drew dark, the clouds were gathering. I had two full days left at home with the children. I wanted to hold onto every minute, but slowly and inexorably events were unfolding. We received a phone call from the sister on Ward D to tell us that Mr Meyer had decided to do an investigation called a Wada test. This, she briefly explained, was to determine which side of my brain was dominant in controlling my speech, understanding of what was said to me and memory. The test would take place on Tuesday, the day I was to return to hospital, but Mr Meyer suggested that we call on Monday afternoon so that he could fully explain the procedure to us. My initial reaction to this phone call was disappointment; my heart sank at the prospect of missing even a couple of precious hours at home. I did not want to go back into that place even for an afternoon. I wanted to stay at home. But I also realised that Mr Meyer's decision to do the test showed just how thoroughly and diligently he was working on my case. I felt that he would leave no stone unturned and no avenue unexplored in his quest to give me 'the best chance of coming through this.'

We rang a doctor friend of ours, who was able to confer with a colleague, a neurosurgeon, to give us a little more information on the test. He also said that with Mr Meyer, I was 'in good hands'. I was glad to have confirmation of what I had already felt. Earlier in the afternoon I had written, or rather dictated to Tony, a note for Mr Meyer. In it I said:

Although I am frightened about Thursday's operation, I will go through it and come out the other side. I will survive this – I'm sure I will. I know that if anyone can do this operation, you can. I trust your skill and judgement.

I wrote this because it was the truth; it was deeply felt and I wanted him to know it, and perhaps I wanted him to know me too. I felt he should be aware that just as he would be there at the end of the operation, so would I. I was certain that he would get me through it, and that he was probably the only person who could do so. Mr Meyer was clearly a very experienced and highly regarded surgeon, but my trust in him arose from more than just that knowledge. It was clear to me that my operation was very risky; however, for me there was little risk involved – if the operation was not attempted, I was likely to die anyway. In a sense, it was Mr Meyer and his team who were taking the risk. I felt that this was not a risk that every surgeon would be prepared to take; it had to be someone who was quite an extraordinary person.

My gut feeling was that Mr Meyer could do the operation successfully and that not only could I trust him, but that also I would be there too. Even though I would be unconscious during the operation, I felt somehow I would play my part in it. In my note I also said:

When I am under general anaesthetic I believe it is likely that, even though I cannot respond, I will hear and take in anything which is said. Therefore I would ask that any comments be positive and realistic, and take into account my dignity and intelligence.

I was not at all sure whether to give this letter to Mr Meyer. I felt perhaps it was presumptuous and arrogant of me to write it, and that it would be inappropriate to give it to him. I was not sure how he would react. In any case, I packed it in my bag, I would take it with me when I returned to hospital on Tuesday, and decide later whether or not to give it to him.

Monday 14 February

On Monday morning, the phone rang. Tony answered, and when I saw his face ten minutes later, I knew something momentous had happened.

'That was Ange. They've got a kidney for Paul! He has just gone into hospital for a transplant.'

Ange's husband Paul had been on dialysis for several years, and recently he had become increasingly unwell.

'She wanted to let us know. She says it's a good sign, that this is going to be a good week.'

I was so moved by this, delighted for them both, and touched by Ange's emotion and kindness – that she should pass on their good news in such a generous and thoughtful way. It was a wonderful and amazing thing to have happened. The timing seemed incredible and it did indeed feel like a good sign, a symbolic and portentous start to an eventful week.

In the afternoon, Tony and I went over to the hospital. I was told that Mr Meyer would see us at about 4.30, but that first I was to have a CT scan and then an electroencephalograph. As I was taken down in the wheelchair for my scan, I felt very cold, and as I sat shivering, Jean, the radiographer, found me a blanket. Then she helped me onto the scanner couch and gently wrapped the blanket round me. This act of kindness and tenderness seemed to me to represent everything that the radiographers gave to me. Their care for patients went far beyond the bounds of their professional expertise. As I lay there in the scanner, snuggled and safe in my blanket, I felt cared for. Even though I lay alone inside the machine with its moving beam of light and penetrating rays, I felt comforted. When I came out, Jean helped me into the wheelchair and tucked the blanket in around me. I thanked her for her kindness.

'You and Pauline have been quite wonderful. I'll never forget the kindness you showed me in September when I had my first scan.'

'Well, I just try and imagine every patient is a member of my own family, and how they would feel.'

I was taken back to the ward, and then Maggie from the Neurophysiology department came to collect me for an EEG. This reading of the electrical activity in my brain would be used for comparison with a reading done during the Wada test the next day.

As Maggie carefully and methodically attached several different coloured wires to my scalp, we chatted, this time not about schools, but about music. Maggie was a keen musician: she had played with the band The Applejacks in the 1960s, and still played guitar in her free time. She attached the other end of each wire to the machine, and all I had to do was to sit there while the waves of brain activity were recorded. She switched on a flashing light for a few seconds and, when the recording was completed, easily removed the wires from my head.

'If you wash your hair, this blue paste will come off easily. When we stick the wires on tomorrow for your Wada test, we'll use a stronger glue which will need to be removed with solvent. I won't be here tomorrow, so Cheryl will do your EEG. But good luck. I'll pop in and see you later in the week sometime.' And Maggie returned me to the ward, where I rejoined Tony.

We sat with a group of patients in the corridor while we waited for Mr Meyer who would come and see us after he had done the Outpatients appointments. It was a very lively group. At the centre was May, an active and outspoken woman in a pink candlewick dressing gown, who, it seemed, could entertain and offend in one breath.

'She doesn't care what she says,' whispered Nora, sitting next to me. 'She's always upsetting people.'

Helen, one of the patients, was given a Valentine's Day card by her husband. 'Here's your Valentine card, love,' he said sheepishly. 'You won't have had a chance to get me one.' he added wryly. The irony was missed by May as she launched her attack first on him, then on men in general.

'Oh, he thinks she should have got him a card. Cheek? How is she going to get you a card when she's stuck in here. Men! Typical!' she snorted.

He refused to rise to this sharp intervention and genially laughed off the personal attack. Perhaps he understood that the sarcastic comments were a result of the fear and anxiety, anger and apprehension that May and all of us felt.

I looked out of the window, at the grey clouds, and the snow, now lightly drifting down. My heart sank, Fearfully, I thought, What if it gets heavier? Maybe I won't be allowed to go home in case I can't get back. And slowly, gently, it drifted down, only just settling on the ground outside. But in my head I saw snowdrifts, blocked roads. 'He won't let me go home in this,' I thought, 'I'll have to stay in. I know, I'll tell him I left my pyjamas at home.' Such a ridiculous thought; it fleetingly passed through my mind and out the other side.

97

'I hope this snow doesn't get any worse,' I said to Tony. He knew the fear in my voice. He felt it too.

May cut through our quiet exchange. 'He'd be mad to let you go home in this. Look at the weather. You should stay here. He won't let you go,' she insisted, wielding her imaginary power like an axe.

'Shut up, you fucking stupid woman,' I wanted to shout. 'I want to see my children. If I don't go home tonight, I might never go home again. Don't even mention the bloody snow. I don't want to hear about it.' But I said nothing. I looked out of the window at the few drifting flakes. Perhaps he would not see them.

At 4.30 Mr Meyer arrived and pulled up a chair near to us. The Wada test, he explained, would involve, first, an angiogram: as before, a radio-opaque fluid would be injected into the femoral artery in my groin, then directed in turn into the cerebral arteries. After an X-ray picture had been taken of these, a barbiturate drug, sodium amytal, would be injected and directed into each cerebral hemisphere. As each side of my brain in turn was effectively shut down, a neuropsychologist would show me words and pictures, then ask me to read and recall them. The aim of the test was to determine which side was dominant for speech and memory. In right-handed people, the left hemisphere is usually dominant, whereas in left-handed people such as me, either side can be dominant for these functions. The results of the test, it was clear to me, would give Mr Meyer more information on which to base his decision on the approach through my brain: it would enable him to work out a path which least threatened these functions. I felt as he prepared for the operation on Thursday, Mr Meyer would miss nothing, and as I felt this, my confidence steadily grew.

'Can I go home tonight? I want to see the children.'

'Of course you can,' he said kindly. 'Could you return by ten o'clock in the morning? That will give the nurses time to ensure you're ready for the test in the afternoon.'

There had been no question of him preventing my going home in what I could now see was just a light dusting of snow. As Tony and I put on our coats and said goodbye to the other patients, May tut-tutted under her breath, and quickly we left.

Once again we took our route of unreality across the city, a route that felt as if it was taken in slow motion: the six o'clock evening traffic in suspended animation; events gathering pace, yet everything around us seemingly at a standstill.

Val and Doris and the children greeted us. The children immediately went off to play a game with Tony and Val. It seemed that the children and I could hardly relate to each other. The world I was in was far away and remote. I so desperately wanted to be with them, but I did not know how. They too wanted to be with me, but I was not the mum I had been six months earlier. The distance between us seemed greater than ever, but perhaps we needed that distance: the emotion of the situation was just too great for any of us to contain. I think the children knew and could gauge and set the terms for what they could cope with, and although I feel that I failed them in many respects by being so preoccupied with myself and not tuning in sufficiently well or sensitively enough to their needs, communication between us was still going on, but at an intuitive and spiritual level. The children had found their way of coping; the love of Tony and the warmth and the practical help of Val and Doris gave them something constant and solid: a scaffolding to hold on to.

At about seven o'clock, there was a knock at the door. To my amazement and delight, it was Judy, my room-mate from hospital in September. I had not seen her since then, although we had spoken on the phone regularly. She had travelled from her home in Worcestershire to the hospital to see me, and on discovering I had been allowed home for the night, had set off across Birmingham to visit me.

It was wonderful to see her and it gave me a tremendous boost on the night before I was due to go back into hospital, although in some ways I felt quite torn. I had ideally wanted a quiet time with the children – but this was not possible in any case: the house was full and we needed and valued the support of Val and Doris. At the same time it was a relief to see Judy: her visit was a distraction and a welcome diversion from the emotional intensity which bubbled just beneath the surface.

With customary humour, she produced a packet of Hob Nobs, a focus of our joking in September, and a magazine.

'Sorry there aren't any pictures of Imran.'

'Never mind,' I retorted, 'I'll settle for Al Pacino instead.'

With her humour, her warmth and her knowledge of what it felt like to be a patient, she gave me great encouragement.

99

'I've a feeling I'm going to come through this.'

'You will, Viv. That day in September was the worst day of your life. But you've moved on since then. This is different. You will come through it.'

By the time Judy had gone, Josie was in bed, and Stevie followed soon after.

I thought this might be our last night at home together.

Tuesday 15 February

It was half-term week, so the children were not going to school or nursery. Still in their pyjamas as we left the house, they gazed out of the window, forlorn and abandoned. The sorrow on their faces seemed to follow me down the road. It was as if I was running away from it, trying to escape their pain, a pain which I was causing and could not take away from them. I could not look back at their faces at the window, nor at the sad figure of Doris supporting such a burden. I had to look forward. I looked down the road with its thin covering of snow. I looked at the houses we passed, familiar but anonymous, and wondered if I would ever see those doors and windows again, or drive down the road again. Already I was displacing my deepest, most frightening feelings onto these inanimate objects. I could only look forward. The only way back was to go forward and to go through. So I looked ahead.

We turned into the Warwick Road, and as we headed towards Birmingham, we passed advertising hoardings, their two-dimensional simplicity standing out against the flat, grey February sky. We skirted the city, became part of the rush-hour traffic, and then headed out up the Dudley Road and across to Smethwick, to MCNN. I wanted to arrive there, but I did not want to arrive. I wanted to drive round and round, pretend I was going to work, or somewhere else, anywhere. But there was nowhere else to go. This was where I was heading, where I had to go, and what I had to face.

So we pulled into the hospital car park. Slowly I got out of the car.

'Shall I get you a chair?' Tony asked.

'No, I'll be okay. I'll walk,' I replied. I held on to his arm and we entered the hospital.

My bed was just as I had left it, but it seemed somehow impersonal again. During the previous week it had become a kind of home, a space that I had claimed and made my own, but over the weekend I had known again my real home, and while I had still felt something of a stranger there, I also knew I did not belong here. But I was ready to resume the role of patient again, and I knew that in doing so, I would find a form of security and safety. Perhaps it was something to do with the way in which, as an institutional inmate, I was severed from my own world, and with that disconnection came a kind of respite, an escape from the sadness I felt when I looked at my children and feared I would be separated from them for ever. Security came too, from the sense of communion with other patients. We shared illness and anxiety, and knew solitude and isolation. We experienced being separated from home and family, and at both a spoken and unspoken level, we could identify with whatever each of us was going through. There were patients on the ward with a range of neurological conditions, but what we had in common was a knowledge of what it meant to be patients, the struggle to maintain a sense of self, to hang on to our individuality in an institutional setting, in the face of potential disability, bewildering uncertainty, precarious reality, and for some of us, perhaps death.

Alice, a patient in the Wendy House, had multiple sclerosis and sometimes used a wheelchair, and we had a long, and very practical discussion that morning on wheelchairs. I had decided that to be confined to a wheelchair was the best I could hope for. It was obviously preferable to dying, and it was clearly a real possibility that if the operation went well, I would be alive but paralysed down the left side. As I quizzed Alice on the subject of wheelchairs, I was trying to prepare myself for this outcome.

During the morning, the neuropsychologist, Robert, came to introduce himself to Tony and me, and to go over the details of the Wada test. He seemed a kind and gentle person, and it was reassuring to meet him. He was not intimidating, and this feeling I transferred to the test itself. While I expected the procedure to be a little unpleasant, I was familiar enough with the angiogram part of it to know that it was tolerable. And it constituted the next step – a necessary and essential stage in the preparation for the operation – so I was ready and anxious to get on with it.

Terry, Mr Meyer's registrar, came to see us. He reminded us of the risks of the operation, and said that the lesion lay largely in the right thalamus: an area of the brain which served, among other things, as a sensory and motor relay station. He said that stereotactic surgery would enable co-ordinates to be taken of the lesion and a precise approach to be made, using external reference points, from a point on my head, through my brain, to the site of the lesion. The aim, he said, was to remove it. Terry gave us a realistic picture of the operation, and also left room for hope. While his style was undoubtedly different to that of Mr Meyer, I felt that together they fully prepared me for what was to come.

Lucia, one of the nurses, arrived soon after, with a wheelchair. She had come to transport me to the Neurophysiology department, where the EEG wires would be fixed to my head in preparation for the Wada test. Tony helped me into the wheelchair, my left leg now having to be placed for me on the footrest. Then he accompanied us as we wound our way along corridors to the small room I had been in the day before. The wires were carefully and firmly stuck to my head, and then when Cheryl, the neurophysiologist, had checked that each one was recording an output, I was taken back to the ward, my colourful 'locks' hanging down behind me.

We arrived on the ward to find Graham, a friend of ours; he had come from the hospital where his work was based to see me, and was then going on to see Paul, whose kidney transplant the day before had been successful.

'Three hospitals in one day,' he cheerfully mused.

'You could take this up professionally, Graham,' I joked. 'Do you like my hair extensions? I asked, pointing to the wires trailing from the back of my head.

Shortly after Graham's departure, I was given a theatre gown and a pair of the inelegant paper knickers I was to wear for the Wada test. When the black trolley arrived, I was helped onto it, and lay there propped up, looking straight ahead. In order to cope with what lay in front of me, my field of vision had already been narrowed. And my emotional field of vision was also restricted: I could only focus on what lay directly in front of me, and could not take in any peripheral matters. Humour and a little self-mockery were ways of doing this. But everything else had to be blocked out. I waved goodbye to Tony and was swiftly wheeled out of the ward, down the long corridor. Then came a sharp turn right and a slower push up the hill. We turned left into the narrow passage leading to the X-ray area, squeezed past the shelves stacked with files, and went left again, stopping outside the X-ray room. Standing by the entrance was Mr Meyer who greeted me courteously and kindly, before I was wheeled into the room.

The X-ray rooms are not dark, and yet they seem dark. This one had a gloomy, cavernous quality; it seemed to be packed with huge, threatening machines, and as I was wheeled in, it was comforting to be met by the radiographers.

'Hello, love. We'll just get you ready.'

Speedily and efficiently, they stuck on heart monitor pads, and fastened onto my arm the cuff of the automatic blood-pressure machine. They cut open the paper knickers and covered me with green sterile cloths, leaving the area of my groin, by the right femoral artery, exposed. The radiologist came in and introduced himself.

'Just a scratch,' he said, as he prepared to inject the local anaesthetic. Like a wasp sting, the needle went into my groin. Then he inserted the catheter; there was a deep pain as the narrow tube was pushed into the artery. I bit my lip and wished I was somewhere else.

'Nearly there', he reassured me, and soon the pain eased. The large black camera was brought down over my chest.

'Breathe in – and hold it', he instructed, as a chest X-ray was taken in preparation for the surgery on Thursday.

Then the heavy camera was brought down over my face, its crushing weight almost touching me. The contrast medium was injected, then directed by the catheter in turn towards each of the main cerebral arteries. As this was done, pictures were taken of the arterial layout of my brain. With each one, hot, crackling images of blood vessels appeared behind my eyes. I could feel them and see them: disturbing and disconcerting flashes of the roadways in my head. I could hear Mr Meyer specifying exactly which pictures he wanted. I understood the importance of his having detailed knowledge of the layout of the blood vessels. He was a very thorough man who left nothing to chance.

The camera was moved away, and Robert, the neuropsychologist, and Mr Meyer appeared by my right shoulder. Robert explained that the drug would be injected through the catheter, and then he would show me some simple pictures, a line drawing of a cat, for example, then ask me to recall what I had seen. He would similarly show me some short words, which I was to read and then later recall.

As the drug anaesthetised the right cerebral hemisphere, I started to feel wonderfully light-headed, a bubbly, champagne kind of drunkenness. I was able to remember, with some prompting, the pictures and words I had been shown. With drug-induced familiarity, I was calling Mr Meyer by his first name.

'You don't mind if I call you Carl?' I asked, with some slight awareness that this was perhaps a little informal.

'Not at all,' he chuckled.

'Oh, I feel really pissed – like I've had three gin and tonics,' I cheerfully mused to Robert, who sweetly smiled.

Mr Meyer re-entered my field of vision.

'No, I don't – I feel like I've had half a bottle of Australian Chardonnay,' I decided.

'That's more like it,' he smiled.

Then the drug was directed to the left cerebral hemisphere. The next thing I knew, Robert was standing on my left, holding the book of pictures and words and asking me to recall what I had seen.

'You didn't show me any pictures,' I drunkenly accused him.

'Yes, I did,' he laughed.

'No, you didn't,' I insisted.

'I did.'

'No you didn't. You did not show me anything,' I protested. I was convinced I had been shown nothing. Even when Robert gave me clues or prompted me, I still had no recollection whatsoever of any words or pictures.

'You showed me nothing,' I teased him. It was far more fun to argue than to accept his word. I could have continued in this way for quite some time. Perhaps I did. I cannot remember.

I can remember, however, an air of fun and merriment in the room, and a sense that I was somehow responsible for this. I had a feeling at the time that, although I could not see them, there were a lot of people behind me at the back of the room. I believe that a Wada test is uncommon, and therefore many staff had come in to observe it. I think I must have sensed I was playing to an audience; I was aware of their amusement, and was enjoying the occasion. Ironically, I was having fun. Absurdly, I felt in control. Paradoxically, while I knew I was facing the possibility of dying, I felt essentially alive. The playful, childlike side of my character was being expressed and I was delighting in this. It was a feeling that seemed to be infectious and pervaded the whole room. The sense that I had of the staff enjoying the humour was a feeling of their participation and involvement, a sense that they were enjoying the fun with me, at my invitation and not at my expense. In this as in so many other ways the staff in the hospital demonstrated their quality of care and their humanity.

Full of fun, mischief and barbiturates, I was returned to the ward. As on the two previous occasions, I had to lie flat for the next few hours to ensure that the punctured artery did not bleed. This was boring and frustrating when I wanted to get up to no good. If I had had my rollerboots with me, I would have whizzed off down the ward, that long smooth corridor crying out to be skated along. Instead, I cheerfully set to work detaching the EEG wires from my head. They were glued on quite firmly and would be removed with solvent, but, before anyone had a chance to try, I gaily prised a few from my scalp, pulling out some hair into the bargain: what the hell! Like a child picking scabs, and knowing, maybe even hoping, that it would horrify the nurses, I became engrossed in my self-appointed task. Barbara, a kind nurse with a sad, almost mournful face, was my challenge. I had been determined to make her laugh for some time, and with the help of the 'truth' drug, I was getting near to success; mixed with her shock when she saw what I was up to was the trace of a smile.

Because I was not allowed to stand, or even sit up to use a bed pan, Kate, a young and highly efficient nurse, insisted I use the 'slipper pan', one to be used lying down.

'Kate, I can't use that. How can anyone use that? Can't I have the commode?' I pleaded.

'No, you must lie flat,' she firmly reminded me. 'You know that,' she added with an implicit appeal to my common sense.

'Kate, you're a cruel and heartless woman,' I accused her. 'She's a cruel and heartless woman,' I repeated to anyone within earshot. She laughed and went off to get the slipper pan. This girl would go far. She was clearly destined to be a sister.

With the persistence of a drunk who thinks they have stumbled on a good line, I repeated this on several occasions. I tried it later on Barbara in the vain hope she might be more easily persuaded.

'Barbara, can I stand up yet? I'm sure I'll be okay. This artery's not going to bleed now. I'm fine.'

'No, you have to lie still,' she insisted.

She was no soft touch!

'Barbara, you're a cruel and heartless woman. You're just like Kate.'

She laughed. Success!

Visitors came and went. Staff regularly checked on me, and I enjoyed giving them a hard time. Pierre, Mr Meyer's houseman, came in and told us that the test had shown the left cerebral hemisphere to be dominant for speech and memory. I was among the minority of left-handed people for whom this was the case. It meant that the better surgical path was through the upper part of the brain, the parietal lobe, rather than through the temporal lobe at the side of the head: the former route was less likely to harm the functions of speech and memory. Even in my still slightly doped state, I knew this was an excellent result; another good sign.

It had been a day of contrasts and contradictions – from its haunting beginning to its light-hearted and uplifting ending. The humour, indeed the whole atmosphere of the Wada test, had been a fitting preparation for what was to follow. It was a preparation not only in medical terms, but also in psychological terms: it provided a useful and helpful means of release, and the sense of exhilaration and euphoria it generated provided a source of energy, an emotional boost that I needed and would draw on. There seemed, however, to be more to it. Reflecting on it all later, I was reminded of seeing King Lear at Stratford, and being struck by the powerful combination of comedy and tragedy in the production dominated by Antony Sher's portrayal of the fool as a twentieth-century clown figure, a Buster Keaton who combined sense and nonsense. The scenes of comic relief offer a release of tension, an interlude before, and a diversion from, the drama of the main event. However, they do more than this: within these scenes lie the key elements of the drama itself. The comedy reflects the same aspects of the human condition as the tragedy, and so it provides not just an emotional release, but is integral to the main action. The Fool is in a unique position to highlight the central issues of the play, themes such as power and identity. When Lear in his

106

madness asks 'Who is it that can tell me who I am', the fool acutely replies, 'Lear's shadow'. It is the fool who embodies and draws attention to the paradox of Lear's position, for it is he who is the wise man who sees the truth.

My experience of the Wada test was not only a time of comic relief, but also seemed to me to encompass many contradictory, even paradoxical, aspects of what it meant to me to be human. Central to this was the feeling that at the point of facing my possible death, I felt so essentially alive and, increasingly, that I was going to live. Confined in a dark, oppressive room and wired up to machines, I felt liberated and free to be myself. At my weakest and most vulnerable, I felt strong. As helpless as I had ever been in my life, I experienced some sense of power and control. In a state that was passive, I felt active, an agent not a victim. Lying there in a position of indignity, I found I had dignity. It was a time of contrasts and of incongruity. At the centre of such precision and order, in the midst of science and technology, lay a redeeming sense of anarchy and chaos. Among the hard, impersonal machines and the menacing black metal, there was human warmth and good humour: the profoundly personal co-existed with the impersonal. Hope lived with fear. In the joy of being childishly silly in such a serious situation. I found not only a way of coping with fear and anxiety, but also a sense of the sheer absurdity of what it means to be human. The Wada test, in the way it contained these universal and paradoxical elements of the human condition, was a fitting prelude to what lay ahead.

Wednesday 16 February

I lay in bed on Wednesday morning, listening to the sounds of activity on the ward. Two of the other patients in the Wendy House were chatting to each other.

'It's so boring in here.'

'Yeah, there's just nothing to do'.

'I wish we had a video or something, I am so bored.'

As I listened to them, I felt envious. I thought, 'I would love to be bored. Oh, for the luxury of being bored. If I didn't have this awful fear, I would enjoy lying here being bored.'

Lucia, one of the nurses, came in to see me. 'Are your children coming in today, Viv?'

'Yes,' I replied. 'They'll be in later.'

Half an hour afterwards, Valerie, the ward sister came in.

'Are your children coming in today, Viv?'

'Yes, they're going sledging with Tony and my sister, and they'll call in later this morning.'

Soon after that, Denise, one of the auxiliaries appeared. 'All right, Viv? Are the children coming in today?'

'Yes, they'll be in around lunchtime.'

'Good.'

They all seemed to be very anxious that I saw my children. It was an anxiety that I did not fully pick up at the time. In fact, I did not register it, or its full significance, until some time later. This was the day before my operation. Some months later, in a moment that made me shudder, I realised that they had suspected, consciously, or unconsciously, that it would be the last time the children and I would ever see each other. But I did not see this at the time. What I saw, and what I felt, was their kindness and concern; they cared about me, and it mattered to them what happened to me. I knew that the staff on Ward D were with me all the way.

Later that morning, Tony, the children, my sister Val and my mother-in-law Doris all came in to see me. The children were bubbling with excitement at the prospect of sledging, but there was also a sharp edge to that excitement, and a great sadness lying behind it.

Josie, my four-year-old daughter, looked at me. Then she said, 'I don't think you're going to get better, mum.' Then she looked out of the window at the snow and the allotments, and she imagined her life without me. I followed her gaze.

'I will get better, Josie.' But at that moment I was not at all sure that I would.

Dressed in her PE teacher's anorak and tracksuit trousers, Val turned to the children. 'Right, kids. Are you ready to go sledging?'

This was met with great cries of excitement and eagerness. I knew the children would have a lovely time with Val; her enthusiasm was infectious, and I knew that with Tony and Val, they would be safe. I hugged them both. I would see them in about an hour. So they departed; I walked over to the window and watched them climb into the car and then drive away.

I rejoined Doris, and we sat and talked. It was so easy and comforting to sit with my mother-in-law. With her, I felt secure, cared for and loved. I knew that she loved the children, and would give all she could to them.

An hour later, they returned. The children and Val were all damp and rosy-cheeked, talking excitedly about their fun in the snow. Tony was genial and good-humoured as ever, but tired and weary; a weariness which came, I knew, not from the outdoor activity, but from the great burden he was carrying, the fear he could not express and the strain he was under.

Val and Doris prepared to take the children home. We hugged each other. We felt each other's sadness but we acted as if this was an ordinary goodbye. I did not know if I would see my son and daughter again. They did not know if they would see me, but somehow we were relieved to bid goodbye to each other, the distance between us the only way we could cope with the pain. It was as if I had unconsciously handed over the children to Val and Doris, as if I was calling on them to take my place, should I die.

Tony and I were sitting quietly chatting when Lucia appeared. Lucia was an efficient and intelligent nurse, attractive and full of life and energy.

'Viv, would you like to come down and see Laurie?' she asked. 'She's had her frame fitted.'

Laurie was a patient who had a suspected brain tumour and, later that day, she was to have a biopsy taken using the stereotactic method: a needle inserted under local anaesthetic with guidance provided by the frame.

Laurie and I had not talked much, but at an unspoken level we had identified with each other, although I did not realise how much until later. She had a lovely, lively family, and Tony had felt a common bond with them; a sense of their warmth and mutual identification.

'Oh, I don't know,' I replied. The frame would be fitted to my head that afternoon, and I was not sure I wanted to see someone who had a metal frame screwed into her skull.

'Come on,' urged Lucia. 'She's fine. She's sitting up in bed chatting away.'

I reluctantly followed Lucia down the ward. Laurie was propped up in bed, the large frame screwed into her head and covered by a green sterile cloth.

'Hello,' I mumbled, half-embarrassed at being called in to witness her discomfort, and also afraid of my own fate being revealed to me. 'How are you? What was it like? Was it okay?' I clumsily asked, my words stumbling out. I did not want to ask, nor did I want to hear an answer. It was unfair to ask, but I was unable not to.

A shadow briefly passed over Laurie's face. 'Yeah, it was okay,' she replied, with dignity and consideration for me. I think she had sensed that I did not really want to know what it was like, and with intuition and kindness, she had protected me. I soon left, and rejoined Tony by my bed.

The interchange reminded me a little of conversations about childbirth. The myth that it is rewarding rather than painful is constructed and perpetuated, and it is only on the initiation of giving birth that we learn the infinitely more complex and subjective nature of the 'truth'. I suspected that this was the case here: in a short while, I would experience my own 'truth', but until then I did not really want to know.

An hour or so later, Lucia rushed in to the Wendy House with a wheelchair and some electric hair clippers.

'They want you down in theatre. They're going to fit your frame, now.'

The request to send me down so soon was unexpected and had obviously taken Lucia by surprise. Me too. I was already in my theatre gown, but my head had not been shaved. She quickly plugged in the clippers, which made a lot of noise, and tugged and tore at my hair, but did not remove any of it.

'They're not working,' she exclaimed in a panic. 'But we've got to get you down there. They'll shave your head down there.' Hastily, with Tony's assistance, she helped me into the wheelchair, and we raced off down the ward.

We arrived outside the theatre area to be met by one of the nurses. 'This is not the patient,' she said. 'It's the biopsy patient we're waiting for.' They were clearly expecting Laurie; my turn would come later. My pounding heart and lurching stomach temporarily settled as we made our way back to the ward. Laurie was taken down to theatre and Lucia went off to find some clippers that did work.

110

She soon returned, then sat me down on a chair in the middle of the room. Strangely, perhaps, I felt very little anxiety at the prospect of my head being shaved. Whenever one of the doctors said to me, 'You'll have to have your head shaved. It will all have to come off,' I replied, 'That doesn't matter. It's the least of my worries.' And I meant it; I had other, more serious concerns than my hair. In fact, while I could see that others thought it would be quite upsetting for me, I almost welcomed it. Having my head shaved was like a preparation for some kind of initiation rite. My bright orange hair was probably one of the last of the images I hid behind.

I sat on my chair in the middle of the room, heard the buzz and felt the tickle of the clippers as Lucia carefully and methodically removed it all. I watched as it fell to the floor: locks of hair, two inches long, mainly bright orange but with grey-brown roots.

When Lucia had finished, I went over to the basin and rinsed the tiny, prickly loose bits of hair from my head. Then I glanced at myself in the mirror, and caught sight of my unadorned self. I looked across at the hair Lucia was now sweeping up. I felt I was moving on. Having my head shaved and not minding was a little ironic. Until I was 32, I had hair so long that I could sit on it. I had talked for years of getting it cut short, but had never been able to do so. Then in 1986, my mother died, and about six months later I had my hair cut into a short, spiky style. Shortly afterwards, I had it coloured orange. I liked it and it had remained that way ever since. I came to realise later that what had been for me a big, but fairly unconscious step, was in fact an outward expression of a profound inner change. When my mother had died, I had finally separated from her and had begun a new stage in the process of growing up.

I saw my bald head and quite liked it, although I thought my ears looked too big. I decided to try on my floppy black velvet hat. Tony got it out of my locker and passed it over to me. I put it on and looked at myself in the mirror. I looked dreadful.

'Tone, do you remember that comedian in the early sixties, Freddy "Parrot-face" Davies?' I pulled the hat down over my head, left my ears sticking out, and did a ridiculous impression of the man who would hold his hand level with his nose and splutter, 'I'm thick up to here.'

Looking bemused and bewildered, Tony made no reply.

Our friend Chris called in. I think it was all quite shocking for her, and probably fairly surreal when I started clowning around and doing my impressions of 'Parrot-face' Davies.

Then the theatre staff arrived with a trolley. I looked at it, gulped and then said, 'Have I time to go to the loo?'

'Yes, of course, love.'

Then, once again, I sat propped up on a black trolley, said goodbye to Tony and Chris, and looked forward. This time I was definitely going to theatre; it was no false alarm. I was accompanied by Sophie, who, as a newly qualified nurse, had yet to observe a frame being fitted. It was reassuring to have her with me as I was taken to theatre, and I focused on what lay ahead.

I was pushed down the corridor leading to the operating theatre, its double doors swung open and I was wheeled straight in, to be met by its gleaming sterility and the sight of several masked figures. The three surgeons were momentarily disguised by their green outfits, face masks and covered heads. Mr Meyer stepped forward to greet me, and then asked me to swing my legs round and sit on the side of the trolley with them hanging down. Pierre stood facing me, and took hold of each of my hands.

'Ah, c'est mon ami Pierre,' I said, as I recognised him. 'Ça va?'

'Pas trop mal,' he replied.

'Meilleur que moi, j'espère,' I commented. Pierre, I knew, was from a bilingual family. Bizarrely, I had initiated this conversation in French, but the prospect of what was to come soon put a halt to my faltering use of the language, and as he held my hands in what was an action of support and empathy, I soon reverted to English.

Mr Meyer was standing behind me and, like an actor who can command a stage with his presence, he was clearly in control. Terry, the registrar, moved forward, holding a long needle.

'Hello, Vivienne. We'll do the front one first. I'll just give you some local anaesthetic.'

The needle went into the centre of my forehead; the sharp, sharp sting seemed to go on and on. And yet I knew this was nothing: a bolt was to be screwed in next. The spike pierced the skin. It was slowly turned. Round and round it went. A little blood dripped down. I closed my eyes. Warm red blood trickled down over my eyes.

'Swab, nurse.'

112

Tighter and tighter. The screw was turned. Pressure was increasing. Tighter and tighter it went. Still more the screw was tightened. I gripped Pierre's hands, clenched them, dug my nails in.

At some point, I started to talk. I talked and talked. I never stopped. With every turn of the screw, I grunted out words. I talked to Terry about bands we had each seen, about Van Morrison, The Saw Doctors.

'The Saw Doctors? At the Humming Bird? Yes, we saw them there too,' he said.

'Yes, they were brilliant,' I replied, drawing on my past enthusiasm. 'It was a great atmosphere.'

Another turn of the screw.

'I like U2 as well. I saw them last summer.' I grunted out each word.

Pierre joined in. 'Did you? So did I. At Wembley. The concert when Salman Rushdie appeared.'

'Yes, that's the one.' This could have been a conversation in the pub except for the way I was expelling every syllable.

By now, Terry had stopped. It was time for the two bolts to go in at the back.

Mr Meyer stood behind me, and to the left. 'Now these will be a little tender,' he warned me, 'because of the angle we need to have the frame.'

A needle went in, just behind my left ear lobe. The long, sharp needle stinging and piercing. It slipped. 'Damn,' he muttered. The icicle-cold liquid dribbled down my neck.

The sharp point went in again; I clenched my teeth. The needle was withdrawn. The spike broke the skin and bit into the bone. A warm trickle of blood slowly dribbled down the left side of my neck. A nurse gently wiped it away. The screw was turned. Tighter and tighter. The pressure intensifying. Words lurched out of me as I continued my 'conversation' with Pierre, and gripped his hands still tighter.

'Yes, I really like U2. Bono's amazing. A bit pretentious, maybe. But sexy.'

I heard a voice from somewhere. 'What was that she said?'

'That Bono's pretentious but sexy,' Pierre quietly replied. 'Who else do you like?' he asked me. 'You play the saxophone, don't you?'

'Yes, a bit.'

'Do you like jazz?'

'Yes.' A short pause. 'I like Prince, too.'

'Oh, Prince.' He seemed surprised. Maybe he thought I was too old.

Mr Meyer was still fixing the bolt into the left side of the back of my head. Twisting and turning the bolt, pushing it in, firmly fixing it so that it would not move. For the shift of a millimetre meant everything. The tighter it was, the more firmly the frame would stay fixed. Precision was everything. There was no margin for error. My life depended on this frame. So with every increase in pressure, I grunted out my words, words of determination. Every syllable of my trivial conversation mattered. I pushed my way through, like a battering ram at the impregnable doors of a solid fortress. I would get through. I would. Never have I known such determination in my life. I was not giving in. I would get through. I would grunt and push and force my way through. I would not give in.

The surreal conversation slowed down. My words were subsiding. Mr Meyer standing behind me on my left, encouraging me. 'Go on, keep on talking to Terry. You're doing really well.'

So I carried on talking. On and on I went. 'What kind of music do you like, Mr Meyer?'

'Oh, music, I don't know. I'm too old,' he muttered. 'I like Black Adder, though.' A slight ripple of surprise at this disclosure passed through the theatre.

He moved across to stand behind my right ear. Once again I felt the scorpion sting as the needle went in. The screw broke through my skin. Turning tighter. Pushing and crushing. Compressing my skull.

'This is not quite the right angle. We'll have to move the two at the back.'

The angle was vital. I knew it was vital. The bolts were removed. Once again they were fitted, turned and tightened, carefully and methodically, turning and tightening, unrelenting, pressure increasing.

Sophie, the young nurse, fainted. If I had been watching this, I would have fainted too. But as it was, I kept my head down, and I kept going. On and on it went.

'Terry, is that one at the front tight enough?' Mr Meyer asked.

'Yes,' I snapped at him. Of course it's bloody tight enough, I thought.

'Okay,' he quietly answered.

114

Finally, it was over.

'You've done well,' he said.

I let go of Pierre's hands.

'Just taking you down to scan, now Viv,' said one of the nurses.

Wheeled along on the trolley. A heavy metal frame screwed into my skull. A feeling of tremendous pressure. Weight. Pain.

We turned into the room housing the CT scanner. My old friends the radiographers were there. The minute I saw them I burst into tears. My body was racked with sobs. Everything I had held in erupted from me. Great, convulsive sobs shook me. And the all-encompassing care from the women there held me. I was helped onto the scanner table, and my head, with its load attached, was carefully placed in position. They did their jobs well, but with their deep humanity, their great love, these women gave me more than could have been expected. They completely took the force of my reaction, stood firm against the explosion of my shock. They allowed it all to come out, comforted and soothed me, became my mothers.

Sophie, the young nurse, was with me again. I felt for her, and I appreciated her rejoining me. She held my hand. While I knew no one would want to undergo my experience, I also knew I would not have wanted to be in Sophie's position. The frame, while it was clearly the means, the only means, by which my life would be saved, bore more than a passing resemblance to an instrument of torture. To stand and passively observe would leave a person feeling helpless and powerless. She or he would witness the pain and torment, but would have no sense of being part of its ultimate intention: to heal. The doctors fitting the frame were not powerless. While they were the ones causing the pain, they were also the agents of its final purpose, its hopefully beneficial outcome. And for me, the patient, the 'victim'? I was not a victim; I, too, was an active participant, playing my own grim part in the procedure. Talking my way through it. But keeping going, all the time keeping going. Gritting my teeth, grunting out my words, I played my part. Mr Meyer was preparing for the operation. So was I.

When the scan was over, I was transferred onto the trolley, where I half-lay, half-sat, propped up, the huge, heavy crown and green cloth on my head. Then I was taken back to the ward. As I was wheeled

115

down towards the Wendy House, I could see quite a large group of visitors waiting for me. I felt quite daunted by this; in my shock and pain, I had hoped for the solace of Tony's quiet constancy and support. I felt a little self-conscious to arrive in this fashion: sitting on my throne like an Elizabethan monarch, wearing my grim, green headdress, my skull-crushing crown.

And yet, the crowd of visitors, overwhelming though it at first seemed, was also a help to me. The determination I had felt during the fitting of the frame had turned into an expression of shock and a need for comfort when I had seen the radiographers. The next transformation was into anger.

'They never told me it was going to feel like this,' I raged. 'I had no idea it would be so awful. Even the local anaesthetic hurt. It all hurt. It was awful,' I shouted.

Friends clustered round us, taking the force of my anger and cushioning Tony's silent shock. Some drifted into the corridor, just outside the room, quietly chatting to each other. It was about six o'clock in the evening. A long night lay ahead of us. We needed their support and diversion. These friends bore the first wave of my shock and anger. I let it out unreservedly and relentlessly; and they took it all. Their own shock, they kept hidden. They had come in to see me the night before my operation – a brave thing to do: they knew how risky the surgery was, they knew I was frightened and that I would be unable to play the usual social games. That I would let it all out, whatever I felt. And they accepted it.

One of the people there was Jean, the mother of Alison, my close friend in Northern Ireland. She was deeply distressed by the sight of the frame screwed into my head. It overwhelmed her. She was here almost by chance: visiting their son in Birmingham, Jean and Bob had wanted to call and see me, and as it happened to be the night before the operation, they had encountered more than they had bargained for. Bob is a calm and quiet man; he kept in the background, while Jean did the talking. As she hugged me, distress poured from her. As her words gushed out, I could feel how much she cared, how she took on my pain; she was engulfed by it, but she was not afraid of it. If she had been afraid, she would have left. In fact, when the time came for her to go, she found it very difficult and painful to leave. She would seem to be about to go, and then hug me again. 'Oh, my dear,' she would say, as she held me tightly. She felt for me as if I was her own child.

'Give my love to Alison when you get back. And give her a cuddle from me,' I asked.

At some point, one of the registrars came into the room. He had a group of students with him.

'And how are you?' he asked benignly.

'Terrible. Awful,' I shouted. 'Why isn't this done under a general anaesthetic? It was awful. I can't believe how awful it was.'

If my friends had caught the first wave of anger, then this was the second, and the poor doctor who had stumbled into the ward was understandably totally unprepared for it. He was clearly taken by surprise, and did not know what to say.

'Well, it's just one of those things,' he mumbled, before hastily beating a retreat.

As the first group of visitors departed, I opened the large box of chocolates Alison's mother had left for me. One by one I stuffed them in, pausing between chocolates to mutter and mumble, groan and grumble.

'This is fucking awful.' Hazelnut Slice. Finely chopped roasted hazelnuts, blended with praline and covered in milk chocolate.

'I hate this place.' Rum Truffle. A double-cream truffle containing Jamaican rum dipped in dark chocolate.

'I'm pissed off with this.' Walnut Truffle. Fresh-cream truffle with finely chopped walnut pieces covered in rich milk chocolate.

'I wanna go home.' Noisette. Praline with brandy and chopped, roasted almonds, coated in white chocolate.

'I'm fed up.' Cherry Truffle. A double-cream truffle laced with kirsch, topped with a glacé cherry and covered in dark chocolate.

'Do you want one, Tone?'

'No thanks,' he replied, as he quietly observed my desperate attempt to find comfort.

'Probably just as well,' I muttered. 'I've eaten all the best ones.'

Two more friends arrived. Stewart and Dee, like everyone else who came that night, had not realised what they would be walking into. And again, like everyone else, they accepted what they found. They took my anger, my shock, my fear and my determination, and held it for me, just for a while. They feared that their presence was intrusive,

117

but it was not at all. I greatly appreciated their concern and their courage.

Then Bernie arrived. I had felt she would come in that evening. I knew that she accepted and understood all that I expressed. It was so good to see her and to feel her support.

Stewart and Dee left, and a few minutes later, Mr Meyer arrived. I was sitting on the side of my bed as he came in.

'And how are you, Mrs Martin?'

I turned on him. The shock and anger I had expressed before was just a starter, a taste of what had been building up inside. With venom and fury, I unleashed my words. 'You never told me it would be like that,' I accused him. 'Why can't it be done under a general anaesthetic?'

'Because it's not good medical practice to do something under a general when it can be done under a local. There's also the problem of scanning someone while they're under a general anaesthetic.'

I looked out of the window to my right and behind my bed. I saw the snow and the fences and the back gardens. 'If I had known what it would be like, I would never have signed for it. I would never have gone through that. I would run away rather than go through that again.' And I gazed out of the window and imagined myself running through the snow, vaulting over fences, crossing roads, running for miles till I rejoined my children.

This onslaught had taken Mr Meyer by surprise. I had turned my shock into a personal attack and made him the focus and the embodiment of the horror that was the frame. Like a child lashing out with fists of rage and fury, I was blaming him. The frame, which was made to his own specification, had become the symbol of all my fear and uncertainty, my physical and emotional pain, the weight and horror of my torment over the last few months and the possibility of my death. It carried all of these meanings and I displaced them onto Mr Meyer. He bore the brunt of my reaction.

'Well, you don't have to have the operation if you find the frame intolerable,' he countered.

I shrank back at this. I realised I had gone too far. The anger which had erupted from me was natural, but it was unfair of me to have directed it in such a way. I became more conciliatory.

'Of course I want the operation,' I said quietly. 'Of course, I do.'

Then he said, 'We all admire you. The whole team. I admire you. You have faced something I don't know if I could face.'

118

I was deeply moved by this. The genuine and powerful exchange between us had been shocking but significant. On the night before my operation, such an honest encounter somehow gave me all the confidence I needed. I knew it was right to give him the letter I had written on Sunday. I asked Tony to get it out of my locker.

'I hope you don't mind. I wrote this note for you,' I mumbled, as I handed it to him.

He opened it and read it. I thought I should explain the last part in which I had asked for any comments made during the operation to be positive.

'I don't mean to imply that anyone would say anything that was unfair. I just mean that I don't want any comments like, "Bloody hell, she's not going to make it",' I joked.

He laughed. 'You've got me,' he said, and folded up the letter, put it back in the envelope, and placed it in his pocket. Then he produced the form of consent for my operation. I could hardly grip the pen or write my name. My signature for the craniotomy was a barely discernible wavy line: the fine line between life and death.

The encounter ended on a light-hearted note. I had made some earlier comment on my Elizabethan headgear, and Mr Meyer picked up the reference with a joke about my Renaissance look, referring to the towelling draped over my head and tucked-in round the sides of the frame to hide it from view. Then he left, accompanied by the sister.

Two of the theatre staff came in to see me, Roy, the ODA and Dr Stevens, the consultant anaesthetist. They were lovely people, warm and kind. I would see them both in the morning when I was taken down for the anaesthetic.

Val, my sister, came in. She had put Josie to bed, and then left the children in the care of Doris while she came over to see me. I knew that with Val and Doris, the children would be well cared for. Val went home and Tony stayed with me. I was exhausted and in some pain and discomfort. There was a long night ahead of me, but I felt that it was the last stage; there was the prospect of an ending and the possibility of a new beginning.

Tony held my hand. I could not find a way to be comfortable. It was difficult to sit; the pressure and weight of the frame was such that it was an effort to hold my head up. I was exhausted and wanted to rest. I tried to lie down. At first, I lay on my stomach and put the front of the frame on the pillow. But as soon as I did this, the frame exerted more pressure on my forehead. I did not know what to do with myself. I was so tired, but I could find no position to lie in. However I lay, wherever I placed my head, the pressure from the frame increased.

Molly, the sister, was very concerned about me. I could see it in her eyes and feel it from her as she took inside her my pain and exhaustion. She helped me to sit up.

'You can't lie like that. Let's try and make you more comfortable.' She rearranged the pillows and propped me up in a sitting position. Molly was wonderful that night. She fussed over me and Tony. She checked on us regularly. There was no question of Tony leaving at the end of visiting time. It just seemed to be accepted that he would stay. The bed next to mine was empty, so he pulled it nearer, lay on it, and was able to hold my hand. He had told Val that he might not go home that night. He could not and would not leave me. 'I'm not leaving you like this,' he told me. No one could have given me the kind of support Tony gave me that long night. Like a solid rock, or the roots of an ancient oak tree, Tony was immovable. The more I leaned on him, the stronger he became; he was truly himself that night. I knew he would have done anything to take the pain away from me, to carry the weight for me. And it was so hard for him that he could do neither of these things.

To observe the suffering of someone we love is agonising. We would do anything to relieve them of it. When my mother was dying, she suffered greatly, much more and for much longer than I was now. The growing, gnawing pain of the cancer worked away at her body. It spread from her ovaries, throughout her digestive system and her liver, and it claimed her body. As she wasted away, devoured from the inside, she was in pain, and she was cold. She lay in Newcastle General Hospital on a hot sunny day, and she shivered with cold. My sister and I held her wasted body in our arms, to try and keep her warm. They wrapped her in aluminium foil – some kind of thermal blanket. I would have done anything to relieve her suffering, to have given her at least some respite. I knew that it was difficult for Tony to watch and to feel so helpless.

I was finding the increased pressure on my head from lying on the pillows was too great. I was exhausted but sleep was out of the question. Molly suggested I try sitting up in the armchair. She helped me to get out of bed, gently and carefully sat me in the chair, and arranged the pillows around me. These afforded me some support, but still my heavy head would loll to one side, pulled down by the weight of the frame. Screwed into my head, the massive burden of the frame had to be borne, however, or wherever, I lay or sat.

Wednesday become Thursday.

Thursday 17 February

At some time in the early hours of the morning, I tried to leave the Wendy House to go to the bathroom. I misjudged the width of my head with its steel attachment, and bumped it in the doorway. The solid side jarred my skull. I was glad then that it had been screwed on so tightly, for if it had altered its position, I do not know what would have happened. But it stayed firmly fixed.

A little later Tony went down to the bathroom. I may have dozed. Then I felt dizzy, cold and clammy. I knew I was fainting. There was no one there and I knew I was losing consciousness. Imprisoned in my steel cage, I was powerless to prevent myself from fainting.

Then Molly appeared, She saw me lolling in the chair. She immediately called for a doctor. 'I think you've fainted my dear. But we'll just be sure.' She looked after me and with great solicitude helped me back into bed.

Tony returned. 'Don't worry,' I told him. 'I'm okay. I just fainted.'

Then a sleepy young doctor arrived. Bleeped at five o'clock in the morning, he had to gather his wits, do whatever checks were necessary, and make sure I was all right.

It was snowing lightly. Just a few more hours to go. Nearly there. Not long till nine o'clock. I hoped the snow would not become heavy. I did not fear the operation but I was afraid that something would happen to prevent it from taking place. What if there was a heavy snowfall? What if the surgeons could not get into the hospital? What if? What if? All I wanted was for the operation to go ahead. It was the only chance I had. And the only way that I could be released from the pressure in my head, or from the vice around it. The frame was my burden; I carried it in a literal sense. But it also metaphorised the weight I had been carrying since September. Ironically and para-doxically it was also the only means by which I could be relieved of the burden I had carried since then.

At about seven o'clock, Molly brought Tony a cup of tea. There was none for me, of course: 'Nil by mouth' hung over my bed. She was going off duty. Her night shift had come to an end. She hugged me and wished me well. 'I'll come and see you when you're on the unit.' I would be taken to the High Dependency Unit immediately after the operation.

'I hope they bring me back here after that. You're all so lovely on this ward.' The staff on Ward D had been incredible. For the last week and a half, they had supported me and encouraged me, with a depth and quality of care that was unsurpassable.

I was given my theatre gown. Tony had a bowl of cornflakes. I gave him my watch. They would soon come. I hoped they would come. So did Tony. I have never been more ready for anything in my life. Never more focused, nor sure. Every part of me. My whole body, my mind, my spirit was ready. I did not feel helpless nor frightened. Just sure. When I had seen other patients taken down to theatre, I had imagined their terror. I had imagined how it would feel when the black trolley arrived and they took you away. I had wondered how they would be afterwards. But most of all, I wondered who they would be afterwards.

The trolley arrived for me and I was helped onto it. I felt no fear. Just certainty. I knew where I was going and I was ready. It was a certainty and a feeling of being prepared that was the culmination of all the emotions and experiences I had undergone since September. Each one was a preparation for the next. There was an order and a meaning to it all. A sense and a purpose. As I was wheeled down to theatre, accompanied by Tony, it did not even cross my mind that I might not survive the operation or that I would no longer be myself. It did not occur to either of us to say goodbye to each other. The sense of certainty underlay everything. While it arose from my intense focusing on what lay in front of me, and was arguably a self protective responsive to a life-threatening situation. I knew it was more than that. It was not a feeling, not an attempt to suppress my fears – they were there and were real enough. The certainty was a deep instinctive knowledge that transcended everything that was going on around me, or happening to me. I think in those few days leading up the operation I was privileged to sense something that was beyond the rational, beyond the way we construct our realities, to see a meaning and a dimension to life I would never have imagined possible. I experienced something that was deeply spiritual and had a glimpse of something that was more certain and more meaningful than I had ever known before.

I was taken into a room, where I was greeted by Roy, the ODA and by Dr Stevens, the anaesthetist, and the rest of her team. A drip needle was inserted in my left hand and small white dots were stuck on the inside of my right forearm. Tony stood by my side, dressed in a gown and a hat.

Roy said, 'Now is there anything you want for when you come round?'

'My glasses. Oh, damn. They're in my locker.' I turned to Tony. 'Make sure they're by my side when I wake up.' I explained to Roy, 'I hate not having them. I feel helpless without them.' I turned back to Tony. 'Don't forget. As soon as they've done this, go and get them.'

'Don't worry, they'll be there when you wake up,' Roy assured me. 'Now can you count to ten slowly?'

'One, two…' Then I knew no more.

What happened during the next six hours is a story for other people to tell. It is Tony's story, who, after he had been told by Roy that there was no need to dash off and collect my glasses – 'She's not going to need them when she wakes up' – had gone to the dining room, drunk coffee, eaten breakfast and written a long painful letter to Steve, his closest friend, who lives in Australia. It is a story for our children, Stevie and Josie, and for Val and Doris, who were watching over them that day. A story for my dad and for our families and friends who thought of me, who focused their love and energies on me. It is a story for the people who sent me spiritual healing, who used their gifts to channel and direct spiritual help to me on that day. And it is a story for Mr Meyer and the team who performed the operation.

The next thing I knew, I was throwing up, my throat felt sore and my head hurt. Tony and Bernie were by my side. I have dim memories of voices in my ear. 'It's out. They've got it all out. Everything's all right.'

I threw up again.

'Hello, Vivienne.' A nurse's voice. I wish they wouldn't call me that, I thought. I hate being called Vivienne.

'Hello, Vivienne,' she repeated. 'Do you know where you are?'

Bloody hell, I thought. I'm in the Midland Centre for Neurosurgery and Neurology, but I'm buggered if I'm going to say that lot.

'Smethwick Neuro,' I said. 'Ward 10'. I had no idea what ward I was on, but she obviously wanted an answer.

'What day is it?'

Shit. I'll have to work this out. I struggled to think. Now my operation was Thursday, so I think it is still Thursday.

'Thursday,' I said.

'Who's the Prime Minister?'

Flippin' heck. 'Er – John Smith,' I replied.

'John Major,' I was corrected. Was this a Tory plot to get us when we were at our most vulnerable? If it was, it had not worked. I had easily forgotten John Major, and opted for the then Labour leader.

'Can you lift your left leg? Good. Well done. Now your right.'

A few days earlier, I had said to Tony, 'The first thing I'll do when I wake up is to try and move my left leg; if I can, then I'll know I'm not paralysed.'

It did not even occur to me, as I obeyed the nurse's instructions, that what I was doing meant that the operation had succeeded. Not only was I alive, I was also not paralysed. But if, as I emerged from the anaesthetic, I was regaining consciousness, it seems to me now that I was not conscious of being conscious. It was a first stage of consciousness – my awareness was of an immediate present, not of a past or a future. I drifted away again. In and out of consciousness I floated, Tony and Bernie's voices drifting across me.

'Oh, I feel sick.'

Bernie held the bowl. I threw up over her hand.

'I expect you're used to this,' I said, referring to her work as a nurse.

'Not from my mates, I'm not.' she retorted.

I threw up again. 'My throat's sore.'

'They'll have intubated you,' she told me. Was that intubated, or incubated. I wondered.

It was question time again.

'Where are you?'

'What day is it?'

'Who's the Prime Minister?'

Lights in my eyes. Pulse. Temperature. Lift your leg.

124

The frame was still on. It would stay in place for another night. If there was a haemorrhage, they would need to get in quickly. So it had to stay in place. The heavy metal tools to undo the bolts were in a bag fastened to my theatre gown. There was a drip in my left hand. I could hear the 'beep, beep' of a machine, some kind of monitor, behind my left ear. 'My head hurts,' I moaned. I drifted off again.

I drifted back. Question time again, or 'Neuro Obs' in the jargon.

'Hello, Vivienne, can you tell me where you are?'

Oh, bloody hell. I can't be bothered. But, like a good girl, I answered, 'Smethwick Neuro.'

Doctors came in to check on me. One was heard to say, 'This is amazing' as I answered the questions, moved my legs.

I am so tired. My head hurts. This bloody frame. The weight. The pressure. I still can't get comfortable, I thought to myself. I did not think, it's over. I'm alive. They got it out. I'm not paralysed. I just thought, I feel sick, my throat's sore, my head hurts.

But there must have been some dawning realisation of my survival, for at some point, Mr Meyer appeared on my right side.

'Hello,' I said. I was pleased to see him. I could not remember if he had already been in. 'I can't remember if I said thank you for what you've done, but thank you,' I said.

He smiled and shrugged his shoulders, I think. I drifted off to sleep.

Friday 18 February

I lay on my back, the frame pressing into my head. As I drifted in and out of consciousness, I played with the thing on my finger. It slipped on and off quite easily. If I allowed it to slip off, the 'beep, beep' from the machine behind me would stop. If I put it back on my finger, the sound would start up again. In a desultory fashion, I toyed with it, flipping it on and off.

'Vivienne, will you keep that probe on your finger?'

Oops, told off. As a child, I was only called Vivienne when I was being reprimanded.

Sarah, the kind and friendly nurse who was responsible for my care as I emerged from the anaesthetic, was no longer on duty. I did not know the names of any of the night staff. I wished Sarah was there. I longed for the nurses on Ward D. I felt desperately thirsty. But how could I ask for a drink when I knew no names. How could I call out 'Nurse, could I have a drink?' It seemed so rude. Names are so important. With them we can reach people, be reached, connect. Without names I was lost. Lost and disoriented. Adrift in space and in time. I had no means of locating myself. It was probably the early hours of Friday morning, but I could not be sure. I had no sense of time. I was just a body lying in a bed, wired up to machines, imprisoned by a metal frame. I felt confined and helpless. It felt as if my only human contact was the torch shone in my eyes and the questions, 'Where are you?' 'Who's the Prime Minister?' 'What day is it?' I had to think very hard about the last one. At some point I realised that it was no longer Thursday, but I could not be certain.

The night went on. A nurse rinsed my mouth with a mouth swab.

'Please could I have a drink?' I asked.

She gave me sips of iced water through a straw. The most delicious drips of water. I could have sipped that water for ever, but a few sips were all I was allowed.

Time went on. Consumed by thirst, I asked, 'Nurse, please could I have a drink?' It seemed so impolite to call out like that. But I could do nothing else. No names and no eye contact. A few dim lights somewhere far off. I lay there. Listening. Longing for voices I recognised. Wishing for the nurses on Ward D. Drifting. Coming and going.

It must be morning. I heard the sounds of breakfast. Someone was asked, 'Cornflakes, love?' The night must be over, I thought. I felt so alone, terribly alone. Lying on my back I could see so little. And so I listened intently to the sounds around me. And then my sense of smell came into play. Someone I recognised was on the ward. That smell. I knew it. It was aftershave. It was Pierre. Somewhere in the distance I heard his voice. Maybe he was coming in to see me. It would be lovely to see a friendly face, to talk to someone I knew. But his voice went away. The scent disappeared. I lay there disappointed. Dislocated and disconnected, I drifted back to sleep.

Sarah was on duty again. Then Pierre and Mr Meyer arrived. They had come to remove the frame. I was glad, but I was nervous. Would it hurt?

Sarah came over. 'Your husband's on the phone, Viv. He's just asking how you are. He wants to know if the frame is still on.'

'It's just about to be removed,' Mr Meyer said.

'Have you any messages for him?' Sarah asked me.

I struggled to put my words together. I felt self-conscious and incoherent as I said in what felt like slurred speech, 'Just give him my love.'

Sarah went back to the phone to convey my message to Tony. Then she returned. Mr Meyer and Pierre set to work on the bolts at the back. There was a momentary tightening of the first one. I tensed and squeaked in anticipation of pain. 'It's all right,' Mr Meyer reassured me, and in fact there was no pain. As each bolt was removed, the pressure eased and Sarah dabbed away the blood. She sprayed and cleaned the three small circular wounds. Mr Meyer indicated to her that he wanted all the dressings changed. As the two doctors departed, Sarah set to work. She had a lovely manner. Even though I was less than 24 hours out of brain surgery, she treated me as a person; she related to me with great kindness and respect. I had a drainage tube coming out of the back of my head. Carefully and gently she placed the dressing around it. Thoroughly and methodically she replaced all of the dressings and then firmly encased my head in a bandage. I was exhausted when all this was done, and now I could lie back. With the frame gone, the weight and pressure finally released, I could at last put my head down. It was tender, but it could touch the pillow. Now I could rest. Relieved and exhausted, I slept.

But not, it seemed, for long. I heard voices. 'We're taking you down for a scan now.' I felt the bed being moved. I lay on it, trying to find my sense of direction as I was wheeled round corners, along corridors and eventually into the scanner department. I have not got the strength for this, I thought. All I want to do is sleep. They lifted me carefully and gently from my bed onto the scanner table. I lay inside the machine. My head was scanned. Passive and dazed, I lay there. I was moved onto my bed again and taken back to the unit. Then, worn out, I slept. Apart from the Neuro Obs – the lights and the questions – necessary checks on my level of consciousness.

A doctor came to administer my intravenous drugs. 'I remember you from the Wada test,' she said. 'I was there'.

I groaned. 'What did I say?' I asked. 'I bet I sounded really silly.'

'No, you didn't,' she kindly reassured me. 'You sounded intelligent.'

It was a little like remembering a drunken night out: it was great at the time but afterwards you cringe and think, Oh hell, what did I say? I bet I made a complete fool of myself.

But I appreciated that she had remembered me, that she knew me a little, even if it was as the 'mad drunken woman from the Wada test.'

I drifted back to sleep again. Tony came in. We cried a little. I think I was starting to realise that I was alive. But I was not fully aware of it. I was still dazed and bewildered. Some information was getting through to me, however. I had been told that what had been removed from my brain was a blood clot. Preliminary investigation had suggested it was not a tumour. I was vaguely aware that this had to be confirmed by a fuller analysis. I think I knew deep down that while things looked good, I could not leap around for joy until the subsequent histological examination confirmed that there was no malignancy. But I pushed this thought out of my mind, for cancer meant radiotherapy, and radiotherapy would be done stereotactically. Stereotactic meant the frame, and I could not bear even the thought of it. I dozed, but as I drifted in and out of sleep, the dreams came. Nightmarish images of frames and spikes screwed into my head. Fear. Dark, shuddering fear. Sharp, searing impressions of torture. Of being trapped. I could not escape from the dreams. As I slept, my mind was working away, attempting to process the shock, the assault it had endured. This was necessary. It was the very beginning of digesting the experience and making sense of it. But it was very difficult. Very hard to do. I just wanted to shut it out. To seal away the memories in a deep vault, never to be opened again.

Doris and Val came in. Val noticed the frame on a shelf by my bed.

'Don't talk about it,' I ordered her. 'I don't want to hear about it.' I was glad I was lying flat and could not see it. It was as if the frame contained all my fear, all the horror I had ever known; and I could not bear to face it, to hear about it, see it or think about it. Not yet, I thought. Not ever.

I think Pierre came in. He had a book with words in large print, four-letter words split in half. I was to try to read them. I do not know whether I succeeded or not. I suspect not. I found it very difficult to make sense of the letters.

Two physiotherapists arrived. Dressed in their white tops and navy blue trousers, they always seemed to move in twos. They told me how important it was to keep my legs moving, showed me how to rotate

128

my ankles and encased my lower legs in support stockings. As soon as they had gone, I went back to sleep. At some point, Mr Meyer came in, but I am not sure when. He asked me if I had done any walking. 'I'm just too tired,' I said. All I wanted to do was sleep. To sleep but not to dream.

Day became night. Sarah was no longer on duty. It was the nameless night staff again. Then, to my delight, Paula, one of the night nurses from D ward, appeared. She hugged me. 'Rita sends her love,' she said. 'We're all thinking of you. A little later Molly called in – Molly who had cared for me and fussed over me the night before my operation. She, too, hugged me. 'Everyone sends their love,' she told me.

'Oh, I hope I go back to D ward when I leave here,' I told her. I felt that the staff on D ward were my friends.

Saturday 19 February

I had some cornflakes to eat. Just a few. They tasted strange. But it was good to do something mundane. Cornflakes were an indicator of morning and of normality, so I wanted to eat them. When my Neuro Obs had been done, one of the nurses asked me if I would like a wash. She took my toilet bag and a clean nightie out of my locker, then filled a bowl with warm water. The feel of the warm, fragrant water and of the flannel on my face was quite wonderful. To be sitting up, feeling fresh and clean, no frame screwed into my head, to be able to look around me felt like freedom, a great precious freedom.

Unexpectedly, Mr Meyer arrived. Dressed in casual clothes rather than his dark suit and white coat, he looked as if he had wandered in off a golf course.

'Good morning, Mrs Martin. How are you?'

'Fine, thinks. I feel great.'

'Have you done any walking, yet?'

'Er, no I don't think so,' I answered vaguely.

'Well, I think we'll give it a try. Now, it will feel something like this. I want you to imagine you're on a ship and it's rolling from side to side.' With a combination of precision and empathy, he described to me in detail how it would feel when I put my left leg down and tried to walk.

129

I swung my legs round and sat on the side of the bed. He took hold of each of my hands.

'Now could you slowly stand up?' he asked me.

I stood up. I was facing him.

'Now, carefully, one step at a time.'

I took a step forward. Then another. He held my hands and took steps backwards.

'You're right. It's just like being on a ship.' I could not feel much with my left leg except for numbness and tingling, but it was clearly taking some of my weight. Slowly he walked backwards, holding on to my hands as I took more tentative steps forward.

'Yes, it's just like being on a ship,' I repeated. I was in a state of almost childlike wonder. Amazed that I was walking again. To have woken up paralysed would not have been unexpected. To be walking was a freedom I had not counted on. But in a way, when I had lain in bed, wired up and catheterised, I had not expected to remain like that. Since emerging from the anaesthetic, I had not thought about it. I had been living mainly in the present, suppressing the immediate past and not anticipating the future, apart from hoping that I would return to Ward D.

I sat once again on the side of my bed. Then he checked my visual field. 'Look straight ahead, focus on the end of my nose. Tell me where you see my finger. Top right, top left, bottom right, bottom left. And so on.'

I concentrated on the end of his nose, and indicated where I saw the movement of his finger. There was in fact a gap in my left visual field, but I was not aware of it at this stage. There had been a sequence to the movements and unconsciously I had detected this and was anticipating the next movement. Mr Meyer realised this almost immediately, and commented to the nurse standing beside him, 'She's anticipating and predicting.' So he changed the sequence, and the gap in the left visual field was confirmed. He advised me that I might feel disoriented and have difficulty in finding my way round, even places that I knew well such as my own home. 'This could be a little distressing,' he told me.

My bed was moved in the afternoon, round the corner and further away from the nurses' station. This was promotion! There was talk of moving me onto a ward nearby for a few days, and then back on to Ward D.

130

I was visited again that afternoon by some of the staff from Ward D. 'There's a place for you, Viv. We've saved your corner in the Wendy House.'

At teatime, I was offered sandwiches. I had no appetite at all. Everything I ate and drank tasted strange to me. But I had started to feel under some pressure to eat. I looked at the plate of salad sandwiches. 'I can't eat those, Tony. You take them. Put them in that bag. I know they're watching to see whether I'm eating or not. Just hide them. I'll pretend I've eaten them.' So, under some coercion from me, Tony removed some of my sandwiches. I did not have the energy to resist more openly the efforts of the staff to get me to eat and I could not be bothered to explain my changing sense of taste, so in this cowardly way, I avoided any confrontation.

The Neuro Obs were continuing and I was getting so used to the questions that when the nurse on duty appeared, I reeled off the answers, 'Smethwick Neuro, Saturday, John Major,' before he had time to ask them. 'Can't you change the questions?' I joked. 'They're getting boring.'

He laughed. 'Okey dokey,' he said. 'Who was the first man in space?'

Mistaking this for a game of Trivial Pursuit, my sister, who was visiting, leapt in with the answer. 'Yuri Gagarin,' she said triumphantly.

As the day drifted to an end, my left side was tingling and numb, my disorientation seemed marginally less, and I was very tired; I was glad to sleep.

Sunday 20 February

My sense of time was quite confused. I would look at my watch, struggle to read it, and ask someone the time, but I found it difficult to assign any meaning to it. During the night, one of the nurses had found me sitting bolt upright in bed.

'What are you doing?' she asked. 'It's two o'clock in the morning.'

'Morning? Two o'clock?' I queried. And I could not work out what this meant. I concentrated very hard on it, puzzled over it, but 'two o'clock' seemed to me to be numbers without meaning. It is only now

131

as I look back on it that I can impose some order and meaning on those days in the unit. Night and day, the passage of time, indeed my whole concept of time, felt as if it had been thrown up in the air and had fallen down, scattered and in disarray.

'Okay Dokey' was on duty again in the morning. He was a very kind, friendly nurse with a good sense of humour. I had woken up that morning convinced I had something to do, that I should get up, get dressed and get on with it. When he came round to do my Neuro Obs, I said to him, 'I must get up. I've got to get moving.'

'Just relax,' he said. 'Have a quiet morning in bed with the Sunday papers.'

Confused and disorientated, I was eventually able to let go of the sense of urgency I had woken up with. But I had taken his remarks at face value and I remember thinking, 'How can I read the Sunday papers? I can't see them properly. I had started to realise there was something different about my vision. My eyes were aching from trying to focus on people I was talking to, and I felt I did not quite know where I was.

After lunch, which I pushed around the plate and pretended to eat, Terry, Mr Meyer's registrar, arrived. He told me that the results of the post-operative CT scan were good, and that I could be moved off the unit.

'Can I go back to Ward D?' I asked immediately. I had hounded and harassed every member of staff with this question.

'Yes, all right,' he agreed. 'So long as there's room there.'

'Yes, there is. I'm sure there is. They told me there was room,' I urged him.

Later on, Okey Dokey returned. 'We're moving you onto D. I've just phoned down and they're ready for you.'

'Yippee!' I cheered. I was overjoyed to be returning to Ward D. The staff on the unit had been very kind, but the prospect of returning to the nurses I knew so well, filled me with delight.

In just a few minutes, we were ready to leave. I said goodbye to the staff on the unit, and with Okey Dokey and Tony pushing the bed, I returned to Ward D. As I was pushed down the corridor, past the armchairs lining the row of windows, I was greeted by nurses and patients I knew.

Okey Dokey parked the bed in my old familiar corner of the Wendy House. I thanked him and he departed. I was happy and relieved to be 'home'. Lucia, one of the nurses who had told me before the operation, 'You will come through it', came down to see me. Before she attended to my Neuro Obs, she hugged me. 'You've done really well. It's good to have you back.'

'It's wonderful to be back. I feel like I've come home.' And I did. I felt relaxed, secure and cared for. The sense of dislocation and isolation just seemed to melt away. I knew where I was. Once again I had my own space – a space which was familiar to me. I was with staff I knew and felt I had strong relationships with. Now the process of recovery could begin.

21 February – 1 March

Tuesday was a special day as Tony brought the children in to see me. I had spoken to them on the phone and heard their voices once again; I could hardly wait to see them.

We had wanted to prepare them for the way I looked, and Tony had told them about my shaven, bandaged head.

I lay in bed and could hear their voices as they approached the Wendy House. Then they came in. Josie was wearing her doctor's outfit, a white coat and plastic stethoscope, and she was carrying Babby, who was appropriately bandaged. As a well-loved panda, most of Babby's fur had worn away, so there had been no need to shave his head. However, a large sticking plaster had been stuck on Babby's forehead, and just to be sure, another had been placed on his bottom.

While it was a relief for the children to see me, it was also a shock. I did not look like the person they remembered; the events of the past few months had taken their toll, and it was still only five days since the surgery. When they saw me, they did not see their customary image of mum, but a shaven-headed figure with waxy skin and tired eyes. It was a tremendous shock for them, but they could see I was alive, and until that moment, this was information they had received second-hand. The process of bridging the gap between us could begin. If they were dazed and bewildered at seeing me, the reverse was also true. I still felt some disorientation and was only just starting to realise what I had come through. The 'miracle' that I was actually alive and also able to walk had not really sunk in.

It was during that week on Ward D that I started to realise just how surprising my recovery had been. I had known on a rational level that my chances of survival were slim. The lesion in my brain had been so deeply situated – a doctor told me when I was in the unit, 'right in the consciousness centre' – that I had not been expected to make such a good recovery. I could sense both surprise and pleasure in the reactions of the staff.

On Tuesday afternoon, I was eagerly looking forward to seeing Dr Anderson, who I knew would be back from his holiday. When I heard his voice rumbling down the corridor, I sat up in anticipation. He came in, surrounded by a group of young doctors and medical students.

'Hello, Trouble,' he said affectionately, then picked up a chair and did an impression of a lion-tamer.

'Hello,' I replied cheerfully. 'Did you have a good holiday?' What I really wanted to do was to hug him, but I decided this was not appropriate.

'Come on then,' he said. 'Let's see you do your tricks.' He checked the strength in my arms and my sense of joint position, then asked me to walk. The expressions on the faces of the junior doctors and students were almost of disbelief – I could feel as well as see their amazement. I do not know what they had been told, but it was becoming apparent to me that the fact of, the nature of, and the speed of my recovery had been unexpected. One day when Pierre came in to see me, he said, 'Your recovery is remarkable, just remarkable,' and as he said it, he shook his head as if he could hardly believe it. It was starting to dawn on me what a narrow escape I had had.

The effects of the operation which were most apparent to me in the first few days were the intensification of the numbness and tingling down my left side and the gap in the left visual field. The tingling sensation was becoming stronger, although I knew I could live with it. The numbness meant that I kept losing my left slipper. As my walking improved and I went down to the day room for my meals, I invariably left my slipper behind, as I could not feel whether it was on or off. My co-ordination on the left side was poor but improving. I had been told that the best way to improve it was to use my left hand as normally as possible. However, when I delivered a spoonful of

134

cornflakes to my left ear, I decided to use my right hand instead. Then I realised that, although left-handed, I had always used my right hand for eating; so there was no need for me to use my left hand in a way that was not 'normal' for me.

My visual field defect meant that I spent a lot of time looking for things. If I wanted something from my locker, I would have to walk round it and look at it from different angles. I had a photograph on my locker of my two children sitting side by side. Yet when I looked at it, I could only see my son, who was sitting on the right. On the left, where I knew my daughter was, there was simply an absence unless I moved the photograph to the right. I found this disconcerting and a little upsetting. The other difficulty arising, I think, from my visual field defect was that I had difficulty in reading. When I looked at print, what I saw was a jumble of letters which I was unable to interpret. I wondered if this was how dyslexia felt. When the menu selection sheets were brought round, someone had to read mine out to me, and do the ticking for me, as I was unable to cope with the print or use a pen.

Other effects of the operation concerned my hearing and my senses of smell and taste. I spent a lot of time listening to my Walkman. However, after a few days, I started to notice an increasing discordancy in any music I listened to. It was as if the sounds, which on stereo headphones are split and delivered separately through each ear, were being processed differently by either side of my brain. The music coming through my left ear was registering in a different key to that coming in through my right ear. Thus when put together the whole piece of music was discordant. I solved the problem while I was in hospital by simply using one earphone and listening to mono radio stations, but I wondered how music would sound when I listened to it on the system at home.

There seemed to be an intensification of my senses of smell and taste. Everything tasted or smelt too strong. I found it difficult to enjoy the taste of any food. Even the blandest of flavours was overpowering: potatoes were too potatoey, semi-skimmed milk was overwhelmingly creamy, and anything sweet tasted so powerful it made me wince. I had no appetite at all, and spent a lot of time at meals simply pushing my food around the plate. I knew the nurses had observed my lack of appetite, and meal times in the day room had started to remind me of

135

school dinners, which I also used to hate. I would try the old trick of hiding one bit of food under another, and trust no one would notice. I could only hope that when I went home, my sense of taste would settle down, and with a greater choice of food, my appetite would return.

The possibility of returning home came sooner than I had expected. On Wednesday Mr Meyer came in to see me. He seemed to be pleased with my progress and to my surprise said, 'We can think about getting you home soon. The physiotherapists need to check you can manage the stairs first.' The prospect of home delighted me, although I knew I was not quite ready yet.

I had felt extremely nauseous for several days, and this seemed to be getting worse, to the point where it made me feel quite ill. Lucia had told me this was probably due to extreme constipation. I had been given codeine phosphate as a painkiller when I was on the unit, and as a result was now severely constipated. Lucia had given me a mini-enema on my return to the ward on Sunday, but this had not helped. As my sickness worsened, she decided it was time for action. She felt that once my constipation was cured, my sickness would disappear.

The time for the enema, the big one, was set for Wednesday afternoon. Some friends of ours en route to London from Lancashire were due to visit that afternoon. I have known Ian since I was 15 and he has always indulged in bowel humour. Tony and I had joked to each other earlier in the day that it would be just my luck if Ian and Susan were to turn up around the time of the enema.

At about two o'clock, Lucia arrived, armed with the enema and a commode, and with a cry of 'Kelly to the rescue', she drew the curtain around my bed. Then, just as she was administering it and raising the foot of my bed for maximum effect, I heard, from the other side of the curtains, Ian's voice. I could only shout, 'Fuck off, Coulson. I knew you'd turn up at this moment!'

'Charming,' he shouted back. 'A fine way to greet a friend.'

Lucia was amazed by this interchange. Ian, of course, was delighted and amused, so the whole undignified experience was logged into the annals of events to be laughed about on drunken occasions.

The enema was a success, and strangely, it seemed to end a lifetime of constipation. Whether it was the enema or the brain surgery, I shall never know, but something changed. While I would not go so far as to recommend brain surgery as a cure for constipation, it certainly did the trick.

With my nausea gone and my strength increasing, I was starting to feel excited at the prospect of returning home. Thursday was a lovely day, a happy day. I received lots of visitors. A group of Tony's work colleagues called in to see me, and it was a wonderful occasion, full of laughter and jokes. Being able to listen and join in the light-hearted and friendly banter was a treat. It was a relief and a release to let go of the seriousness of the past few months.

That night, the realisation which had been gradually dawning on me for the past week seemed to finally reach me. Suddenly, I started to feel, I'm alive. I'm actually alive. I've got a future. I can be part of my children's future. I can live my life. I thought of the summer, which seemed to me to be just around the corner, and I was able once again to envisage my part in it. For the last few months, I had had to face the nightmarish prospect of my family carrying on their lives without me. Everything in my life had seemed to be shutting down. Now, in contrast, I could see vistas of possibilities opening up in front of me, and I knew that I could live my life and would not be excluded from the lives of others. When I thought of the future, I could include myself in it. I felt happy, ecstatically and euphorically happy. So happy and excited that I could not sleep. I lay in bed wide awake for most of that night, and I could see a future.

The next morning, Pierre came in to see me. 'On Wednesday, Mr Meyer said I can go home soon,' I said excitedly. 'Just as soon as the physios have checked my use of the stairs.' Arrangements were made for my discharge, and it seemed I would be going home that day. Excitedly, I got dressed, packed my bag and waited to see a physiotherapist. I had not expected to be going home quite so suddenly, but I could barely contain my delight at the possibility of it.

Tony and I waited all that afternoon until the physiotherapist eventually saw me and checked that I was safe to use stairs. I was now waiting to have my discharge confirmed by Mr Meyer, who was in theatre. At about six o'clock, a phone call came down from theatre. It seemed there had been some mistake; I was not to go home. One week after my operation was too soon. I understood this. I had been

137

surprised that 'they' had planned to let me out so early. But, at the same time, I was bitterly disappointed not to be going home. My expectations had been raised, my anticipation of leaving and my excitement at the prospect of it had reached fever pitch. Fully dressed, my bag packed and after sitting around waiting for several hours, I returned to my bed. I sat on it and sobbed. I cursed doctors, hospitals, anything I could think of. I felt as if I had been lifted up in the air and then smashed down onto the ground. Once again, I was confined to the Wendy House. I gazed out of the window at the allotments which had carried all my misery and fear during the last three weeks. I gazed through another window at the back gardens and fences which had represented my need to escape. And I looked out through the windows opposite my bed and saw the car park, the hospital drive and, to the right, the main entrance of the hospital. How many times had I looked longingly at those doors and dreamed about leaving? Well, it seemed I would look wistfully at the exit for a few more days.

Before my operation, I had identified with other patients and gained a great deal from the shared understandings and sense of mutual support. In some ways, and with some patients, this was still true, but in other respects, I seemed to have changed. I was not aware that this was happening, but as I started to look outside the hospital, to a future and a life, I was also beginning to distance myself from some patients. While I could listen and share the concerns of patients with conditions which were different to my own, I was unable to offer any support to anyone who had undergone anything even remotely similar.

I spent some time with Esther, a patient who had Alzheimer's disease. She seemed to me to be deeply distressed and needed to talk. I know nothing about Alzheimer's disease, but it seemed to me as if she was locked into her depression. As soon as she had expressed her sadness and offloaded some of it, she had no memory or sense of having done so. Therefore, she was right back to where she had started, and needed to express it all over again. She seemed to be trapped in an ever-repeating cycle of sadness, and seemed to need a matching cycle of counselling and support. I was glad, indeed privileged to spend some time with her: it meant a lot to me to be able to give some support and find a role for myself.

At the same time, however, there were patients whose concerns I felt unable to share. Two patients were, I knew, waiting for biopsy results. Neither of them openly expressed their fears about this, but I knew such feelings were present. And I just did not want to know. While I had been given the all clear by the surgical team who had removed the haematoma from my brain, and told me that it was not a tumour, but a malformation of blood vessels, I knew that full clearance and reassurance could only come after a more rigorous histological analysis. And if this analysis revealed malignant cells, then I would need to undergo stereotactic radiotherapy. The slight possibility that it could still be cancer, and the thought of the frame, produced such terror in me that I shut it out, I could not contemplate it, and, I think, because of this, I shut myself off from close involvement with certain patients.

My main feeling was that I wanted to get out of the place, and the raising of my hopes on Friday made me realise just how much I wanted to go home. I was told that I would probably be able to go on Monday, but I did not allow myself to think about it. When Tony and the children come in to see me on Sunday, I played it down. I did not want to raise the children's expectations, just in case they were to be dashed again. I went to sleep in my hospital bed on Sunday night saying to myself, 'I will not be going home tomorrow.'

On Monday morning, Terry came to see me. 'You can go home, Vivienne,' he told me.

'Yes!' I shrieked with delight. I raced up the corridor and grabbed the phone. I spoke to my sister. 'Tell Tony to come and get me. I want him to bring my jeans and my denim shirt. Oh, and tell him to bring my big coat. It looks cold outside.' After I had delivered these instructions, I returned to my bed, and gathered together my belongings.

Then Pierre and Mr Meyer arrived, and my discharge and departure were confirmed.

'Thank you for what you've done,' I said to Mr Meyer.

'Just keep on doing as well as you have been doing,' he told me. And Pierre nodded.

By the time Tony arrived, I was dressed and ready to go. I hugged the nurses and thanked them for their care. We thanked the doctors again as we passed them in the corridor. And so I left Ward D. Then I stepped out through the hospital doors. It was not a dream. I was leaving the hospital. I would be well again. I wore my big coat but not my hat. I carried it in my hand. I did not mind my shaven head. I had nothing to hide.

We climbed into the car. The old familiar car, scruffy and like a dustbin, evidence of the children – discarded papers and toys – strewn over the back seat. I was going home. Home to my children. And a future.

On Tuesday 1 March, I woke up in my own bed. When I went downstairs, I put on Bob Dylan singing *New Morning*, and listened as he sang, 'So happy just to be alive underneath this sky of blue'. While this was indeed how I felt, I knew my recovery, particularly my emotional recovery, would be a little more complex. But at least now I had the chance to embark on that recovery.

PART FOUR

March 1994 – September 1995

EMERGENCE

March and April 1994

In *A Leg to Stand On*, neurologist and writer Oliver Sacks describes how an accident on a mountainside in Norway caused him to lose the use of a leg for a while. In this moving and thoughtful account he writes of his experience of being a patient, and of the difficulty of emerging from sickness and confinement into the outside world. He recounts how, on his last night in hospital, his 'unconscious self contrived a near accident' in an attempt to sabotage his discharge from hospital. At a conscious level, he felt eager to leave, but at the same time, the prospect of relinquishing his dependent status was frightening. He then found that such acts as his own were common among fellow patients. I could identify with his reluctance to relinquish the care and the 'cherished-infant status' to which he had become accustomed. He writes of himself and his fellow patients, 'We wanted, consciously, to be weaned, but unconsciously we feared and tried to stop it, to prolong our special, pampered status.'

While I recognised these feelings, my own near-discharge and subsequent disappointment circumvented any subconscious desires to remain in hospital. Ultimately, the temporary setback was helpful and served as a preparation for returning home. When I finally left hospital, I knew that I was ready to move on. But at the same time, I did feel frightened and extremely vulnerable: in fact, the first thing I did on arriving home was sit down, burst into tears and say to my sister, 'I just want to be looked after.' The prospect of emerging from a state of utter dependence and powerlessness was daunting. Physically, I was very weak, still a little disoriented, slow to think and to react. Emotionally, I was in a state of shock. It was as if my every

143

sense, my whole self, had been battered and beaten and I could hardly begin to take in, or make sense of, what had happened to me. I was dazed, and as vulnerable as I had ever been in my life. In a way, I felt more vulnerable after my operation than before it. While I was in the midst of the experience, in the throes of the struggle for my survival, my head was down, my teeth were gritted and every ounce of strength I possessed had been needed to enable me to survive. And psychologically, I had drawn on and used every means of defence available to me. While it was happening, while I was going through it, I was not standing outside the experience, nor reflecting on it, and in fact I was barely capable of reflecting on it. I was living it, and instinctively focusing on coming through it alive. Now that I was emerging from it, my defences fell away. I was weak and childlike in my need for comfort and care.

As had been the case all along. I was in the fortunate position of receiving enormous support from family and friends. On the practical and emotional level, there were reservoirs of support to draw on, and it was given freely and unreservedly.

In this still dependent state, I could not imagine how I could ever again function in the outside world. And in the first few weeks after leaving hospital, all I wanted was the safety and security of home, family and close friends.

It was a kind of regression, a retreat into the womb-like security of home, a retreat that I needed to make. For it was only in this safe environment that I could work through the initial stage of accepting the reality of what had happened to me, of accepting not only the facts of the experience, but the meaning of it. This initial phase of my psychological recovery would require not only an intellectual acceptance, but also an emotional acceptance, a recognition of the depth of the trauma. In fact it was only after I returned home that I started to realise just how difficult it had all been, and in some ways still was. The flash of realisation that I was alive, the euphoria I felt on the Thursday before I left hospital and my delight at coming home, settled and faded. Now, I could hardly begin to think about what had happened to me. I could not wear the pyjamas I had worn in hospital nor tolerate the smell of the soap I had used there. Anything, any small reminder of hospital, would make me shudder. I could not imagine being able to see the place again, to smell it, or to feel its atmosphere.

144

It became in my mind a symbol of fear and torment. I knew I would have to go back as an outpatient for scans and follow-up appointments, but I could not imagine, at this stage, how I would cope with these visits.

As I started to become aware of my vulnerability and to recognise the grim reality of what I had experienced, I was plunged into a dark hole of depression. I would say to myself, 'But I'm alive. I should feel happy.' But I did not feel happy. In his song *I'm Alive*, Jackson Browne sings, 'I want to lose my sorrow and be free again.' This was exactly how I felt. But I did not know how I could do this. I felt miserable and desperately sad, as if I was in a dark tunnel from which I could not escape.

My GP Dr Gabriel, called to see me one day, and as I told him how desperate I felt, he listened carefully and then said in a quiet and thoughtful way, 'It sounds rather like bereavement.' His words, which were spoken with great empathy and perception, showed me that he understood what I was experiencing, that he recognised the validity of these feelings, and also that he regarded them as necessary, as part of the process of emotional recovery. As soon as he said this, I realised it was true. From my own experience of bereavement after the death of my mother, and in my work as a bereavement counsellor for Cruse, I knew that the stages of mourning have to be worked through. There are no short cuts. The reality of what has happened has to be accepted and the pain of the loss has to be experienced. Anything that allows the bereaved person to suppress or to avoid their pain will ultimately prolong their mourning and prevent their recovery. When Dr Gabriel said this to me, I thought, 'That's it. He knows. He understands. He's right. The only way out of this dark tunnel is to go through it, to feel my way, to experience every slow and painful step. There is no short cut and no escape hatch. There will be light at the end of this tunnel, but I will only reach it by working my way along it, by sliding my hands along the damp and slimy walls. I will stumble and fall, but I will keep on feeling my way through it. And I will get there. Slowly and painfully, I will get there.'

It was a great relief to realise that my depression was natural, and was indeed necessary, a part of the journey I had to make if I were to recover emotionally from the experience.

145

I was greatly facilitated in this aspect of my recovery by the support I received from others. For example, a friend who is also a counsellor called to see me. I was feeling desperately low and as if I did not know where to turn. Seemingly out of the blue, Anne arrived, and it felt almost as if she had sensed my great need. She was able to help me to express something of my sadness and confusion, but also to remind me that this was a natural and normal reaction to what had happened, that it was all right to feel this way. I was extremely fortunate at this time to have such quality of support from so many people. Their recognition and validation of my feelings would, I knew, enable me ultimately to move on.

It had seemed to me when I was in hospital that there was an enormous need for counselling support, and I knew that there were many patients who would need this kind of help both in hospital and later, after their discharge. But sadly, though inevitably, such support has a low priority even though it may in the long term prevent depressive illness.

While everyone I came into close contact with was caring and supportive, there were, of course, those who had difficulties in their reactions to my situation and in the way they responded to me. For example, if I answered the telephone, I would on occasion feel the disappointment or the awkwardness of someone at the end of the line when they heard my voice rather than Tony's. They had rung out of kindness to asked about my progress, but it seemed it was difficult and daunting for some to actually ask me how I was, almost as if they were intimidated by what had happened to me. It reminded me a little of the classic experience of the bereaved person whose neighbours cross the road. It seemed that some were afraid of making genuine contact with me, as if they were embarrassed and almost in awe.

Psychotherapist Susie Orbach has written extensively on the emotional illiteracy which prevails in westernised societies. She writes, 'By upholding the cultural and private values about restricting our emotions that we have assimilated into our codes for living, we relegate an understanding or facility with emotional life to the periphery of conscious experience.' It seems to me that the cultural context in which we acquire language, and the resulting limitations this imposes on our ability to express our own feelings in an authentic way, make it difficult for many of us to have the confidence to try to respond genuinely to others. Consciously, we may fear upsetting someone, or we may be afraid of appearing foolish or inarticulate, but *un*consciously we may be shielding ourselves from our own unacknowledged emotions and unexpressed pain. In 'protecting' others, it is often ourselves we are trying to protect. However, while I could understand why people might feel uncomfortable with me, at times I felt impatient and intolerant of it.

Another reaction I encountered was the 'well, at least you're alive' response. I did not find this helpful; I had in fact said these words to myself, and they had not been of any benefit. While I would remind myself that this response also came from the difficulty we all have in unravelling and recognising the complexities of our own emotions, I would still feel frustrated. However, I would agree with them, nod and say, 'Yes, at least I'm alive,' but what I felt like saying was, 'Well, at least *you're* alive. It doesn't mean that you don't get pissed off at times.' I knew I was lucky to be alive, and thankful for it, but I did not see why I should be any more grateful for it than anyone else.

My physical progress was steady and gradual. I was extremely tired, and for the first two months after leaving hospital I slept a great deal. I would sleep for about ten hours a night and also take a nap in the afternoon: my sleep was deep, restorative and healing.

Over this period, there was considerable improvement in my visual field defect and I was gradually able to read again, although I would occasionally neglect material on the left side of a page: for example, if I was looking at the newspaper to see what was on television, I would automatically miss the listings for BBC1 on the left, then realise and read them later. I would often bump the left side of my body and had a string of bruises down my left leg. I am not sure if this was the result of my not seeing something on my left, or whether it came from a slightly impaired sense of my own 'leftness'. Perhaps this amounts to the same thing – I do not know.

There was an occasion when I was sitting in an armchair, my hands resting on my lap. My daughter was perched on the left arm of the chair and then suddenly fell off. I had not realised, but my left arm had floated away from my knee and knocked her to the floor. I wondered if the gap in my left visual field, and indeed my sense of what was happening on the left, together with a temporary loss of awareness of the position of my left arm, had caused this limb to go

147

its own way. It was as if for a few moments my arm did not know where it was. I found this incident quite disconcerting. It was difficult to explain to Josie what had happened, and that I had not intended to send her flying.

My hearing seemed to become normal once again. The discordancy I had experienced when listening to music on my Walkman gradually disappeared as I listened to music on the system at home. The two separate stereo channels were discordant at first, but after an hour or so seemed to merge into an harmonious whole. It was as if the two sides of my brain, which had been working separately while they were receiving the signals through the headphones, were now able to work together and make harmonious sense of a piece of music.

The intensification of the tingling continued. It felt, and indeed still feels, like a fine pins-and-needles sensation. There is a constant low level of tingling, which increases in response to activity: any action which requires co-ordination such as walking or using my left hand, touch, reading, thinking spatially, logically, or mathematically, experiencing or remembering strong emotion.

I had been told that this intensification of my symptoms was likely but when it first started, I felt a huge sense of panic. I did not know what was going on in what I perceived as this hole in the centre of my brain. I imagined blood vessels leaking, and as I had no real physiological understanding of the reason for the increase in the tingling, I had a great fear that something would go wrong, and at times was convinced that something was indeed going wrong. I could not take my health for granted, and could not imagine being able to do so ever again.

Just before Easter I started receiving physiotherapy. The purpose of this was to improve my strength, co-ordination and sense of touch. I started exercises to strengthen my left side, and to improve my gross and fine motor control. From throwing and catching balls and bean bags, to moulding plasticine and picking up lentils with my finger and thumb, my co-ordination gradually improved. With my eyes closed, or my hand in a 'feely' bag, I would attempt to distinguish a range of objects by touch alone. Then, in describing their size, shape and feel, and confirming or correcting this by looking at each object, I would rebuild connections and relearn something of the nature of the world we perceive with our sense of touch. Initially I was unable to tell the difference between, for example, the feel of a pen and an apple. My sense of joint position, which is, as I understand it, the internal, almost unconscious knowledge we have of the position of our limbs, was still slightly impaired in my fingers. So in holding a pen or an apple, I had little idea of where my fingers were, and consequently, of the size or shape of the object. In addition, my sense of touch was impaired, and the strong tingling I experienced when feeling something seemed to distort and confuse the impression I received of it.

Sensations of hot and cold were present but not very acute or precise, and so I had to be very careful when cooking. If, for example, I was lifting something out of the oven, my hand would often unknowingly slip from the oven gloves, and I would touch the hot tin or metal shelf. The feeling of burning was slow to reach me, and by the time I reacted to it, I had burnt my fingers. I learnt to use my eyes as much as possible so that I could see the position of my fingers and avoid this happening.

There was gradual improvement in these areas, and, though still limited, my fine motor control became a little better. However, I had considerable difficulty in writing with my left hand, and could not, for example, carry a cup of coffee safely in that hand.

I was aware of a slight change in my visual/spatial sense. When I was in the High Dependency Unit, I had been warned that I might have difficulty in finding my way around. In fact, any impairment in this area was quite minor. On one occasion, for example, I was travelling with a friend, and when she asked me to give her directions, I found that I had some difficulty in visualising our route – a route which I had known reasonably well. Similarly, finding my way through a crowd when out shopping was quite daunting. I had to concentrate very hard in order to work out and negotiate my way around people. And I would often lose things because I could not picture where I had left them.

For a while, my concept of time seemed to be slightly disturbed. For two or three months, I had a sense of events rushing towards me. I would know, for instance that we would be doing something in three weeks' time, and then suddenly the event would be upon me. It was as if I had lost the sense of what three weeks felt like. I was not easily able to estimate time. Normally, we know approximately what five minutes or an hour feels like, and for a while, I seemed to have lost

149

that knowledge, that feeling of five minutes or an hour. However, gradually this improved.

The sensory disturbance which I found most difficult to cope with, however, was the intensification of my senses of taste and smell. While I had been aware of this in hospital, and had experienced some slight change in taste even before my operation, I had rather assumed that it would improve after I returned home. But I soon discovered that virtually everything I tasted was too strong. Just as in hospital, bread was too 'bready' and milk was too 'milky.' Food which in the past had provided pleasure and comfort, as well as sustenance, could now make me recoil in horror. Every taste was excessive, would shock me, and feel almost like a slap across the face, then a heart-shrinking disappointment. I would have a memory of how something had tasted, and an expectation based on the memory. And every time I ate something, my assumptions would be challenged and my memory disabused. While I knew that on the scale of awful things that could have happened to me, this excess of taste was relatively minor, it actually felt like a huge and devastating loss. I would try to eat, because I knew I had to, but it was an effort. Not only was there no pleasure in eating, there was actually displeasure. Food was unpleasant and felt like a punishment.

Food, Susie Orbach writes, is the 'primary form of relating for the first few months of life,' and as feeding at this time usually takes place within the intimacy of the mother–child relationship, 'the mother's presence is always implicit in food'. I could never have imagined learning the psychological truth of this as an adult, or in such a direct and painful way. We can all talk glibly and easily about 'eating for comfort', but to have this comfort and pleasure replaced by such a repellent experience was deeply distressing. What was most difficult was not knowing how long this would continue. In fact, in its extreme form, it only lasted for about six weeks, and then gradually improved over the next 18 months. However, during that initial period, I had no way of knowing that the 'hyper-taste' would not go on for ever. If someone had said to me. 'In six months, it will be better,' I would have found it easier to live with, but in those first few weeks, I did not know this, and feared that I faced a lifetime of such horror and deprivation.

I existed on a diet of skimmed milk, cornflakes, poached eggs and vitamin pills. I had a particular difficulty with anything sweet, but found that I could eat raw cooking apple, which tasted to me like very strongly flavoured sweet eating apple. However, by Easter there was some improvement and my diet, although still limited, was extending. In fact on Easter Sunday, I decided to try chocolate for the first time. Some friends had given me an Easter egg. Tentatively, I put some in my mouth, and to my delight found that I was not knocked sideways by the taste; the excruciating and overpowering sweetness I had expected did not mask the flavour of the chocolate. I could not say that I actually enjoyed the taste, but at least it was a step forward.

As my physical recovery steadily progressed, I gradually emerged from the pit of gloom into which I had descended in March. However, in order to do this, there were areas of my experience which I was somehow forced to come face to face with. The first of these was the frame. I had not thought about it, and had very consciously suppressed thoughts of it when I was in hospital. In fact, when I was on the unit, I said to someone, 'I don't think I'm ever going to be able to think about this or come to terms with it.'

'Don't. You don't have to. Suppress it. Forget it,' she replied.

'Yes,' I said. 'You're right. I think I'll have to.'

But in the back of my mind, I knew that some day I would have to face the experiences of the last few months. I knew that ultimately I would find it more difficult to suppress these memories, and that if I did avoid facing them, they would return to haunt me in unconscious forms such as flashbacks or nightmares. At a personal level, and through my work in counselling, I knew that traumatic experiences have to be re-entered and relived in order to be fully digested. Then, their shock can be assimilated and one can move on. In order not to be claimed by what had happened, I would have to re-enter, reconstruct and eventually claim something from the events of the last few months. This, I knew, would take some time, would happen at its own pace, and at a combination of conscious and unconscious levels.

The work on post-traumatic stress syndrome pioneered by psychiatrist Gordon Turnbull has shown how vital and effective this kind of debriefing is in preventing future physical and psychological problems. And again, I was extremely fortunate to be in a position to work through my experiences closely supported by friends and family, and also to have friends with counselling skills and experience who could recognise and validate my need to make sense of events.

151

I was also fortunate in that, while I had only moved into the field of counselling relatively recently and had limited experience, I had at least acquired some of the knowledge which would legitimate my way of dealing with events. I knew in an intellectual and a professional sense that it was ultimately an effective and therapeutic way of handling my situation.

However, despite being forewarned, the first time I relived the fitting of the frame took me completely by surprise. I have no memory of what provoked it, but suddenly I seemed to re-enter the experience. I was sitting in the kitchen with Tony and Doris, his mother, and I started to talk about it. As I went through it, my words came out in sobs and grunts.

'Don't talk about it. Don't think about it. It does no good,' Doris advised. But there was alarm in her voice as well as kindness and concern.

'It's all right,' Tony reassured her. 'It's good. Viv needs to do this. It will help her.' Tony calmly and quietly supported me as I relived and described the experience. As my words gradually subsided, I knew this had been a small but significant step towards recovery. I was aware that it would happen again, but that on each occasion its force would diminish until eventually it would hold no power over me.

May and June 1994

The next occasion on which I relived a painful experience again took me by surprise. It should not have done. I should have expected it, but, ridiculously, I was totally unprepared. On 17 May I was due to go to the hospital for a CT scan. It would be my first visit since I had left in February. Strangely, and unusually for me, I had not thought about the scan: I had neither prepared myself for how I might feel at the sight or smell of the hospital, nor had I anticipated the scan itself or its meaning.

The weekend immediately before had been a delight and a distraction. An old and dear friend, Steve, on stopover from Australia, had visited us. We had not seen him for 13 years, and the time we spent with him was so special that I did not think about the scan.

On Tuesday morning, Bernie kindly took me over to the hospital. While I was not conscious of feeling strongly nervous about the visit, there must have been powerful *un*conscious undercurrents. After a

152

plain scan was done, I was brought out of the scanner and given a contrast injection, before being sent back inside again. This mirroring of the first scan I ever had, in which the swelling had been discovered, followed by a contrast scan, produced a feeling of terror in me. As I lay inside the scanner for the second time, a tidal wave of panic rose up inside me. I became convinced that the plain scan had revealed a problem which had necessitated the contrast scan, and all the feelings of isolation and of separation, the fear of permanent separation from those I love, came flooding back to me. The scan following my admission to hospital in February also came flashing back into my mind. The feelings described then, the 'forever faraway, never to be part of their lives' feeling which I had suppressed that day, returned and claimed me. It took me completely by surprise, seemed to come at me from behind and grab me by the throat. I lay still in the scanner, but as the table slid out and the radiographers helped me down, I sobbed, 'Something's wrong. I know something's wrong.' They were kind and reassuring, but I knew that there was nothing they could tell me until the results had been read and interpreted by the doctors. I would have to wait.

Bernie and I sat in her car in the hospital car park and I cried. I had not expected to feel this way. I should have prepared myself for these feelings, but since coming out of hospital in February I had suppressed and denied many painful memories, and inevitably they had resurfaced, then erupted.

'Would you like to go back into the hospital, perhaps onto Ward D, see if we can find someone we can talk to, perhaps Pierre, or one of the nurses?' Bernie asked me.

'No, I just want to get away,' I replied. 'Let's go.' Partly, I was worried about appearing silly or neurotic, but also I was experiencing an echo of my need to escape in September and February.

The whole visit seemed to echo and to mirror previous events and feelings. In fact, there was one small, but unconscious action of my own which I later realised was a mirror image of something I had done in November 1993. As Bernie and I got out of her car on our arrival at the hospital, for no apparent reason, I showed Bernie a bruise on my left leg. I was not aware of it at the time but I now think this may have been a subconscious flashback to the occasion in November when I had made the bruise on my arm the focus of my feelings.

153

So Bernie took me home, and as I was still very anxious and convinced that there was something wrong, she rang Mr Meyer's secretary on my behalf and explained the situation. We were told that Mr Meyer would receive the pictures in a few days' time and that she would pass a message on to him. Until then, I knew I would have to wait and to live with my fear as best I could. On the one hand, it seemed an irrational fear, one which I knew was triggered by unpleasant memories. I knew that I was making good progress and that there seemed to be no obvious signs of deterioration. But on the other hand, I also knew that it was quite rational not to take anything for granted. I had done well *so far*, but after such a major operation, it was reasonable not to assume too much.

A few days later, I received a phone call from Mr Meyer's secretary to say that he had seen my scan pictures and had left a message to be passed on to me that there was 'nothing amiss' and he would see me in June when my follow-up appointment was due. I greatly appreciated the message: it meant that I could push my fears aside for a while.

When I returned to the hospital in June, I saw Pierre and Mr Meyer, who confirmed that the scan had revealed no problems. The histology reports had shown no abnormal cells, nor tumour growth. When I was told this, I said to Pierre, 'Well, I'd sort of assumed this was the case, that if there had been any malignancy, you would have got in touch.' In fact, when I thought about it afterwards, I realised that I had not assumed this in quite such a cool and rational way. What I had actually done was to push the possibility of malignancy and all it meant right out of my mind. I had suppressed and denied these thoughts. If I had been told that the histology had revealed a 'neoplasm' – cancer, I would have been stunned for I was totally unprepared for bad news. I was in a very different frame of mind by this time compared to my psychological state of readiness in January and February.

I was given further explanation at this appointment of my tingling sensation. It seemed that the nerve cells in the thalamic region, the main site of my operation, had gradually changed. Nevertheless, the pins and needles I was experiencing were a mild form of this thalamic syndrome. It could have been far worse – the chronic and intractable pain I had been warned about. While I find it at times intrusive, I know I can live with it.

At around this time, Tony bought *A Leg to Stand On* by Oliver Sacks. As he started to read it, he would say, 'Hey, there's something in here about loss of visual field,' or read out a passage on 'proprioperception', the body's sense of itself and its position.

'What's that? Let me see.' I exclaimed, and before Tony had time to finish the book, I claimed it from him. And I devoured it. I found it one of the most powerful books I had ever read; the right book at the right time. In it were not only explanations of phenomena of which I had some experience, though little understanding, but it was also a gripping and moving story, a personal account of a deep and disturbing experience. Here was a book written by a doctor who knew how it felt to be a patient, who could truly understand how bewildering, how isolating and how frightening it was to be cast into the world of sickness. He knew both as a neurologist and as a patient how precarious our sense of reality is. He understood the loss of confidence in oneself as an independent adult person, the fear of the 'bustling, callous, careless, hugeness of the world'; he knew how trapped we can feel by our limitations, and particularly by our own perceptions of our limitations. I found I could identify with many aspects of his experience, and as I read the account, I felt, I am not alone.

While in many respects I found the book reassuring, I also found it disturbing, since it confirmed what I had already suspected: that what we believe to be objective reality is at least partially subjective and is neurologically and neuropsychologically determined. To that extent it is not external nor constant, it is perceived. I had experienced the subjectivity of what is real, and knew how precarious those perceptions were. When I had inadvertently knocked my daughter off the arm of the chair, I was at first bewildered. My 'reality' had been that my left arm had been resting on my knee. So whose arm had knocked her to the ground? Surely not mine. For a while eating had been transformed from a pleasurable experience into one of shock and deprivation, and my sense of taste was still not back to 'normal'. So, if my 'reality' had been so easily and unexpectedly altered, how could I be sure that it would not happen again. If my perceptions were so dependent on my neurological state, a state which I now knew was uncertain and could not be taken for granted, then I could not be sure that what appeared to be real was constant or unchanging. All I could

155

do was to recognise and learn to live with this precarious and uncertain state of affairs.

July 1994–September 1995

Throughout the summer of 1994 I developed an enormous thirst for the knowledge which would enable me to understand the origin of the swelling in my brain and help me make sense of the experience. I had asked many questions at my appointment in June and also at an appointment at Dr Anderson's clinic in July. I needed to understand what had happened so that I could feel reasonably sure that nothing of the sort could happen again. I say 'reasonably sure' because I am aware that there can be no absolute assurance and no guarantee of continuing health for any of us.

Through my questions and some reading, I came to understand that what had been in my head was a cluster of blood vessels, a 'cavernous angioma', which at a foetal stage had developed wrongly; a sort of spaghetti junction of veins and arteries which had lain there to no ill effect for most of my life, but which was intrinsically weak and at some stage in adult life was likely to short circuit and to bleed: a time bomb waiting to go off. I could draw some reassurance from the fact that I had been so thoroughly and frequently scanned and X-rayed that any other time bombs lying in wait would probably have been detected. The swelling had been completely removed, and with limited damage to the surrounding area, so while I could take nothing for granted, I could be fairly certain that I was well again and would continue to be so.

However, I have to accept that my fear of anything of this sort ever happening again cannot be entirely rationalised away, and is something that I have to live with. Whenever I have a scan or a follow-up appointment, I know that it will produce fear in me: echoes of past emotions as well as new apprehensions. All I can do is to acknowledge and express such feelings, and then try to live my life *as if* I am safe. Perhaps this is what we all do for most of the time: we live, we have to live, as if we can take life for granted. There seems to be a fine line between being aware of how precious life is and having the luxury of taking it for granted.

What I had experienced was more than just an intimation of mortality. I feel that I came face to face with the possibility of dying, and it seems to me now almost that I *had* to face that possibility in order to survive. If I had not confronted death, I could not have turned away from it. When Brenda, the healer, told me that I would be well again, she was showing me that there was a chance for me if I wanted to take it. In the months between then and the operation, I came to realise at the very deepest level that I wanted to live, and becoming aware of this determination within myself meant that in February 1994 when I was offered the possibility of surgery, somehow I was in a position to take advantage of it: it meant that I could go into the operation with resolve, and with a certainty whose source was largely spiritual that I could come through it alive. The spiritual healing, the skills of an exceptional surgeon and his team, and the quality of care I received from a committed and compassionate hospital staff, all combined to give me that chance of survival, and I feel that each of these factors made a significant contribution to my recovery.

I am very curious about what took place during the operation. Not only would I like to understand what happened in medical terms, but I am also interested in what happened beyond the realm of the physical. I know that the spiritual healers were asking for and sending healing to me. Brenda told me that she channelled and directed spiritual help to me and to the doctors. When I came out of the anaesthetic, and was answering the Neuro Obs questions, I can remember one of the doctors expressing some amazement at my level of consciousness so soon after the operation. I was a little bemused by this, for although I was conscious, I was initially not aware of being conscious. When I expressed some vague degree of surprise at his reaction, he shook his head in bewilderment and said, 'Well, we were right in the consciousness centre of your brain.' It is strange for me now to remember this conversation, which took place, I think, just a few hours after surgery.

One of the questions which remains with me is, 'Where was I during the operation?' I know this is a ridiculous question. Obviously I was propped up on an operating table, anaesthetised for six hours, while a plate of bone was removed from skull, my brain was exposed, and along a track through to its centre, a haematoma was carefully excised. While this was going on, I was simply an inert and

157

unconscious physical presence. And yet somehow I feel there was more to it than that. The questions 'Who was I, where was I when it was happening?' may well be asked of anyone who is anaesthetised, but seem somehow more pertinent when it is one's brain which is undergoing surgery. Such questions may have arisen for me from a need not to feel left out, a self-centred and arrogant desire to have been a participant in the operation. This need for active involvement was certainly something I felt from quite early on in my illness and was not a feeling I could easily relinquish.

It is possible my need to be proactive was a small factor in my recovery. I went into the operation as prepared for it as I was able, and I feel now that although I was unconscious during the procedure and 'knew' nothing about what was going on, at some level I was present and played a part in the proceedings. I also feel that the spiritual healing was in some way connected with this. If I regained a level of consciousness which was surprising so soon after the operation, I wonder if it was because in a sense I never really went away; my spirit, my essential self was present throughout. I may not have possessed a sense of self – I had no awareness of self – but I feel that at a psychological and spiritual level I was an active participant, and that my body and soul were one and were working together.

I have written of a certain emotional distance which had developed between the children and me in the months leading up to the operation, and of how I was unaware of it at the time. It is something that I have found very difficult and painful to admit to. My only excuse is that I was focusing so intensely and instinctively on surviving that I was not conscious of it happening. And while I have some understanding of the psychological mechanisms which caused this, and am aware that it could happen to anyone in a comparable situation, it is something which I deeply regret. My love for my children lay at the very core of my desire and my determination to live, but I was slow to recognise the way in which I had handed them over to other carers. For a while, I was physically unable to be part of their daily lives, to pick them up from school, for example, and friends and family had kindly provided this practical support. However, as I became stronger, I was able to become more involved in the routine aspects of their lives. Nevertheless, while we had maintained warm and affectionate relationships, I think it was necessary for me to recognise the distance which had developed, and to understand why it had occurred, before the gap could be bridged. This happened very gradually and, for me, very painfully, but a new depth has developed in our relationships. Like many children, Stevie and Josie are extraordinarily perceptive, genuine and honest. They too have needed to reflect on the experience, and when ready, to talk about what it has meant to them. They both possess an emotional maturity and integrity which I find astonishing and salutary. I have learnt, and will continue to learn, a lot from them.

In February 1995, one year after my operation, it was snowing and the schools were closed. The snow, which was the first we had seen since the previous winter, seemed to trigger a memory in Josie. She started to talk about the day she, Stevie, Tony and Val had gone sledging, the day before the operation.

'I was happy and sad that day,' she told me. 'Sledging was great. I had a lovely time. But I was sad too. I wished you were with us. And I was frightened. What I was frightened of most was that I would only have one grown-up to look after me, and that would be daddy.'

'Yes, I know, Josie. I was frightened too, frightened that I might die and not be part of your lives.'

'That's it,' she said. 'That's it. I thought you were going to die.'

I could feel her relief as she said this. The huge fear that she had carried in her heart for so long could at last be named and we could all acknowledge it. As Stevie, Josie and I sat and hugged each other, we cried and talked about naming our fears and of how it helps to make them smaller. As the children talked about the events of the past year, and as I listened to their words and heard their feelings, I realised how much they needed to express it all. Josie questioned me closely and in great detail about the 'thing' in my head, and as she was doing this, I became aware of how frightened she was that it could return, and I realised that I had not given her enough information and explanation to help allay those feelings. Not only had I underestimated her ability to understand what was happening, but I had also taken for granted that she could accept that the 'thing' in my head had completely gone. I had not realised that she needed knowledge and understanding, just as I had needed it, if she were to have the chance to put her own fears into some kind of perspective. As I answered her questions as clearly and truthfully as I was able, I think – I hope – it helped to reduce her anxiety.

159

Over the last year, my recovery has progressed steadily in all areas. In the summer of 1995, I had a visual field check as requested by the DVLA at Swansea, the outcome of which has meant that I have resumed driving. The day I received the telephone call from Swansea giving me the good news was also the day I realised I could run and jump. A close friend, Jenny, was visiting me, and as I put the phone down and shrieked with delight, I jumped up and down, then ran across the room to hug her.

'Do you realise,' she said, 'you have just run?'

I had not been aware that I had done it or known that I could do it; it seemed that in the sheer spontaneity of the action, in the instinctive doing of it, I had overcome my perceived limitations. The occasion reminded me of Oliver Sacks's rediscovery, after his injury, of 'spontaneous, thoughtless walking'. He writes, 'All of a sudden, I remembered walking's natural, unconscious rhythm and melody.' I had experienced a similar liberating discovery a few months earlier when I had been dancing at a party and had realised that there was a smoothness and fluidity in my movement that was not quite present when I walked. It was as if there had been a connection between the music and my own kinaesthetic sense, and that this had enabled me to move my body in a natural and instinctive way, unhampered by my perception of myself as someone who moves awkwardly and a little unevenly. So now it seems I can drive, I can run and jump, I can dance or swim. Perhaps my roller skates will see the light of day once again.

I still get very tired indeed, and this limits what I can do. I have to pace myself, think ahead and rest when I need to and when I can. Energy is a precious resource which I have to use judiciously and selectively. I have to prioritise: I cannot, for example, do something unimportant in the morning if I know I will need the energy to do something of greater priority later in the day.

The tingling sensation continues and will probably always be there: I do not like it, but I know I can live with it. My sense of touch is present, though distorted by the tingling, and my fine motor control is better than it was, though slightly impaired. This together with my tiredness has meant that I have not yet resumed playing the saxophone. As I was having considerable difficulty in writing with my left hand, I switched to using my right, a transition which I found to be fairly easy, perhaps because, as the Wada test had shown, I was not strongly left-handed. In fact, the whole of this account has been written with my right hand, and I now use it fairly naturally for writing.

Between September 1994, exactly one year after the discovery of the swelling in my brain, and February 1995, I started to write in a haphazard, disorganised and tentative way about the whole experience. These first attempts were vague and fairly illegible scribblings on scraps of paper, but by February I had started to use my right hand, and felt a need and a readiness to work through what had happened in a systematic and detailed way. This has involved re-entering and reliving events and feelings, and from that I have tried to reconstruct the experience. In re-creating and attempting to find some coherence and meaning in what has happened. I think I may be finding a way of claiming something from it all, as opposed to being claimed by it.

One of the ways in which I have coped with being ill has been to turn inwards, to contract and to shut down peripheral areas of my life. As I become stronger and more mobile, it is time for me to turn outwards and to expand. Emerging from sickness and dependency into the big, bold casual world outside is difficult and daunting. I feel vulnerable and fragile, but, as I take tentative steps into the world of work with a few hours of teaching, I am starting to feel I am moving onwards.

The last time I visited MCNN for a check-up, the building seemed smaller to me: the place which had for a while loomed large in my mind as a symbol of fear and isolation seemed once again to be modest and unassuming, but at the same time, unique and quite, quite special. I feel great affection for this hospital which has represented so much to me: not only difficult experiences and painful feelings, but also compassion and hope, community and humanity. As the hospital closes, I feel for those who work there and share something of their sense of loss.

Two years after I was told that there was a swelling in my brain which might not be accessible, I am alive and learning what that means. One year after that diagnosis, I wrote on a scrap of paper:

It has been a year
of discoveries
of connections
of cataclysmic explosion
the big bang.
Minute particles
emanating from the source of light
heading back towards that light
separate and belonging
reflecting and connecting.
In paradox and contradiction
lie understanding and perplexity.

Sometimes I can make no sense of what has happened, but at other
times I feel I have been privileged to glimpse a meaning and an order
which I would otherwise never have known. In that I have been
fortunate.